MENOPAUSE:

What No One Talks About!

By Sharon Brown

The Book Chief

Published by The Book Chief Publishing House 2023
(a trademark under Lydian Group Ltd)
Suite 2A, Blackthorn House, St Paul's Square,
Birmingham, B3 1RL
www.thebookchief.com

Book Cover Design: Sharon Brown
Editing: Sharon Brown
Typesetting / Proofreading: Sharon Brown
Publishing: Sharon Brown

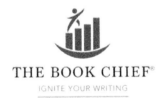

THE BOOK CHIEF®

IGNITE YOUR WRITING

Table of Contents

DEDICATION 11

ACKNOWLEDGEMENTS 13

INTRODUCTION 15

MIDLIFE ACCEPTANCE 17

   Winning Poem of the Kettering Literary Festival 2023 17
   by Sharon Brown 17

CHAPTER 1 21

  EMBRACING THE CRONE 21
   By Amanda France 21
  HOT MESS SELF-HELP 23

CHAPTER 2 27

  BEYOND BIOLOGY, MY WALK TO FREEDOM 27
   By Andrea Hochgatterer 27

CHAPTER 3 35

  RELIEF OR RUIN, HRT'S NIGHTMARE 35
   By Cat Robinson Armor 35
  PROGESTERONE MADE JAYNE FEEL SUICIDAL. 35
  OESTROGEN WAS CAUSING DONNA'S MISERY! 38

CHAPTER 4 43

  FEELING LESS PORN STAR & MORE MENOPAUSAL MONSTER?.. 43
   By Christine Wright 43
  EFFECTS OF ALCOHOL ON MENOPAUSE 45

CHAPTER 5 51

  MENOPAUSE, WOMEN AND WHALES 51
   By Elle Bright 51

CHAPTER 6 56

  TESTIMONY OF FECUNDITY 57
   By Ellie LaCrosse 57

CHAPTER 7 63

  MOVING THROUGH, NATURALLY 63

By Femke Williams 63

CHAPTER 8.. **68**

WHAT IF HRT ISN'T FOR ME?! 69
By Hannah Charman 69
1 – ALWAYS START WITH SELF CARE 70
2 – CHECK IN WITH YOUR MIND 70
3 – LET HERBS HELP! 71
PULLING IT ALL TOGETHER 73

CHAPTER 9.. **74**

MENOPAUSAL ROLLERCOASTER 75
By Helen Helliwell 75

CHAPTER 10.. **81**

MY MENOPAUSE EXPERIENCE 81
By Jo Howarth 81

CHAPTER 11.. **89**

THE POSITIVE POWER OF YOUR MENOPAUSE 89
By Jutta Wohlrab 89
BALANCE YOUR BODY 90
EMBRACE YOUR SECOND SPRING 91
TAKING IT FURTHER 93
YOGA 93

CHAPTER 12.. **97**

GET ACTIVE, FEEL GOOD, EMBRACE MIDLIFE 97
By Lisa Chadwick 97
HORMONE BALANCE AND BONE HEALTH 99
WEIGHT MAINTENANCE 100
BALANCE AND MOBILITY 100
ELEVATE YOUR MOOD 101
ANXIETY AND DEPRESSION 101

CHAPTER 13.. **105**

BACK FAT AND JELLY WOBBLES...................................... 105
By Rachel Young & Cat Robinson Armor 105
NEEMA'S STORY (AGED 48 IN PERIMENOPAUSE) 106
WHAT WE DISCOVERED 107
HOW WE WORKED WITH NEEMA 108
KEY 1 EDUCATION... 108
KEY 2 PSYCHOLOGICAL HEALTH 109
KEY 3 PHYSICAL HEALTH 110
KEY 4 CULTURE AND BELIEFS 110
KEY 5 RESOURCES 111

THE OUTCOME 111

CHAPTER 14 112

MENTAL HEALTH, TRAUMA AND MENOPAUSE........................... 113
By Rachel Young.. 113
WHO IS AT RISK?... 113
I DON'T KNOW WHO I AM ANYMORE 114
A TIME FOR CHANGE 115
UNBURDENING YOUR MIND AND BODY....................................... 115
THE CLEARING-OUT PHASE 116
YOUR TIME TO UPGRADE 117

CHAPTER 15 120

SHE'S HOTTER THAN HELL! 121
By Rita Preston.. 121

CHAPTER 16 129

A FASCINATING PHASE 129
By Sharon Brown.. 129

CHAPTER 17 136

HELP! MY WAIST HAS DISAPPEARED 137
By Sue Copeland.. 137
OTHER POTENTIAL REASONS FOR PUTTING WEIGHT ON AT THIS STAGE OF LIFE
INCLUDE: 137
NUTRITION DURING MENOPAUSE.. 138
Nutrition/Hydration Tips: 138
INTERMITTENT FASTING / TIME RESTRICTED EATING...................... 139
EXERCISE 140
EXERCISE TIPS: 140
SLEEP - CAN SLEEP AFFECT WEIGHT LOSS? 141
STRESS 142
The relationship between stress and weight 142
HERE ARE SOME LIFESTYLE TIPS FOR REDUCING STRESS: 142
MINDSET 143
Six tips for improving your mindset: 143
IN SUMMARY: 144

CHAPTER 18 147

THE "JOYS" OF MENOPAUSE AFTER 50..................................... 147
By Susan Beesley 147

CHAPTER 19 155

A HOLISTIC APPROACH TO POST MENOPAUSE WEIGHT GAIN .. 155
By Susan Beesley 155

CHAPTER 20 163

THE ROLE OF 'INFLAMMAGING' IN MENOPAUSE 163
   By Suzanne Laurie *163*
INFLAMMATION, AGEING AND GENDER.................................... 164
ADDRESSING INFLAMMATION 166
TOP ANTI-INFLAMMATORY FOODS:.. 166
TOP ANTI-INFLAMMATORY LIFESTYLE HABITS 168
   Regular moderate-intensity physical activity:.................... *168*
   Prioritising quality sleep:.. *168*
   Stress-reducing practices:... *168*
   Maintaining a healthy weight:... *168*
   Limiting alcohol consumption: *169*
   Staying hydrated: *169*
   Avoiding environmental toxins: *169*

CHAPTER 21 .... **171**

MENOPAUSE: ONE OF MANY MIDLIFE TRANSITIONS.................. 171
   By Suzanne Laurie *171*
LOSS IN MIDLIFE 172
WHAT IS RESILIENCE? 173
CAN YOU BUILD RESILIENCE? 174
WHAT DOES RESILIENCE LOOK LIKE? 175
AND THE REALLY GOOD NEWS?.. 176

CHAPTER 22 .... **178**

FIGHTING THE MIDLIFE ODDS TO PERFORM AT YOUR BEST 179
   By Tabby Kerwin *179*

CHAPTER 23 .... **184**

SEX AND POO – BREAK THE TABOO!....................................... 185
   By Trudi Roscouet *185*

CHAPTER 24 .... **190**

HOW CAN YOU EMBRACE MENOPAUSE? 191
   By Yvonne Dodd *191*

EPILOGUE... **197**

REFERENCES... **199**

ABOUT THE CREATOR OF THIS BOOK **201**

SERVICES **205**

THE BOOK CHIEF PUBLISHING HOUSE 205
MO2VATE MEDIA 206
THE SPEAKERS INDEX 207

Dedication

This book is dedicated to women all over the world who suffer in silence through menopause and to those who have lost their lives because of it, whether through suicide or related illness.

Keep shining a light on this topic whenever you get the chance and educate as many women and men as possible into the effects this can have on women's health, physically, mentally and emotionally.

Acknowledgements

I'd like to acknowledge the women who have shared their vulnerabilities, truths and experiences within this book in order to educate others to the symptoms, effects and coping strategies.

Thank you to Amanda France, Andrea Hochgatterer, Cat Robinson Armor, Christine Wright, Elle Bright, Ellie LaCrosse, Femke Williams, Hannah Charman, Helen Helliwell, Jo Howarth, Jutta Wohlrab, Lisa Chadwick, Rachel Young, Rita Preston, Sharon Brown, Sue Copeland, Susan Beesley, Suzanne Laurie, Tabby Kerwin, Trudi Roscouet

I'd also like to acknowledge all the women who work in Women's health whose mission it is to help those struggling through midlife and this ever-changing landscape of issues surrounding menopause.

Sharon Brown (The Book Chief)

Introduction

In creating this book, my main aim was to educate other women going through or just starting menopause symptoms.

I knew the ladies who wanted to participate in this would have some challenges to share but also some great input in terms of coping and, at times, a more holistic approach rather than HRT.

Some of the topics discussed here are rarely spoken about and may be seen as taboo to some, i.e. sex drive, constipation, use of alcohol etc., but these are all challenges faced and are essential to recognise and discuss. Sharing and talking to others will make you feel less alone, and you'll understand that every woman has some symptoms that are similar but also unique ones too.

My menopause journey has been challenging and awakening in different ways, as many women within these pages will also highlight in theirs. If I had known more when I was starting, it might have made my journey a little easier, and if I had a book like this, it would have brought comfort knowing others were feeling the same way.

Our hope for this book is that you read it, share it and learn from it. Reach out to the women here who can help you, even just for a simple chat to understand what you can do.

Just remember, you never have to face this on your own…

Sharon Brown (The Book Chief)

(Please note, that all opinions are the individuals Authors' own research unless references have been shared in our Bibliography at the back of the book.)

Midlife Acceptance

Winning Poem of the Kettering Literary Festival 2023

by Sharon Brown

Each morning I rise from my comfortable bed
The to do list is planned for the day ahead
Lifting my phone, I scroll through the posts
Then head downstairs for my tea and toast

My life has changed from much younger days
Working for peanuts, a challenging phase
I started a business more as a dare
But it's turned into something that makes me care

My forties arrived with upheaval and hell
Going round in circles, in life's carousel
The menopause hit and I'm hot and I'm cold
But with confidence and sass, I dare to be bold

The wrong side of 50, but so far so good
the up and the downs, the pain and the moods
The last few years have changed my focus in life
I'm now an entrepreneur, mentor, business owner and wife

Four decades have gone, but I'm happier now
No ego or pride, but also no WOW!
I look in the mirror, another line has appeared
A grey hair, a dimple, it's everything I feared

Each line tells a story of each passing year,
Adversity, truth, failure and fear
For the years there was struggle, there was also a plan
no self-doubt allowed, told myself that I can

―

I started a business for women alone,
we talk every day, online and by phone.
I attempted a man hub but that just fell short
the silence was deafening so best to abort

My ladies are great, they're funny and bright
They're very supportive, they don't even fight
The teamwork impressive, their skills even more
We all work together, we're all at the core

So don't be disheartened when you think life is shit
Everything changes... I used to be fit!
Your path can be written to suit your big dreams
I know it is hard, but not as it seems

Your life will improve with wisdom and age
Your business will boom, you're no longer caged
Enjoy your forties, they go by so fast
Always look to the future and forget your past

I'll leave you now with an encouraging word
You're no longer young, you're just an old bhurd
But with class and finesse, you still look the part
You're gorgeous inside, SO FULL OF HEART!

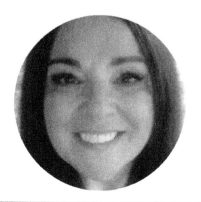

AMANDA FRANCE

AMANDA LIVES IN A VILLAGE IN YORKSHIRE WITH HER FAMILY AND BORDER TERRIER, MIA. SHE WENT TO UNIVERSITY IN SHEFFIELD, HAS LIVED ABROAD AND WORKED FOR VARIOUS BLUE CHIP ORGANISATIONS IN THE UK. AMANDA RETURNED TO HER BELOVED HOME COUNTY, WHERE SHE ENJOYED THE COUNTRYSIDE, NATURE, LIVE MUSIC AND THE YORKSHIRE NATURAL WIT.

SHE IS A FULLY QUALIFIED THERAPIST IN PRIVATE PRACTICE, AN ACCREDITED MEMBER OF THE BRITISH ASSOCIATION OF COUNSELLORS AND PSYCHOTHERAPISTS (BACP) AND AN ACCREDITED PROFESSIONAL REGISTRANT OF THE NATIONAL COUNSELLING AND PSYCHOTHERAPY SOCIETY (NCPS). HER FIRST CO-AUTHORED BOOK WAS "THE SECRETS OF 99 SUCCESSFUL WOMEN".

AFCOUNSELLING.CO.UK
AMANDA@AFCOUNSELLING.CO.UK

Chapter 1

EMBRACING THE CRONE

By Amanda France

As I sat across from my counselling client, I looked down at my shoes; it was not a normal occurrence, but my brain was trying to figure out how this ground-floor office could have an inferno beneath it. The heat rose swiftly up my legs; I was using all my heightened senses to detect any whiff of smoke, and then my vision blurred.

What was going on? I removed my steamed-up glasses casually, but inside I was confused.

I professionally ended the session on time, and when I escorted my client out of the door, I felt a slick of perspiration on my entire body, drying in the crisp winter air. I had experienced my first hot flush!

I soon discovered Peri-menopause takes no prisoners; it rampaged like a rebellious coup in my body. It cared not for the time or the event; it seemed to take delight in steaming my glasses, plastering my hair to my forehead with sweat whilst sending rivulets of the aforementioned, to sting my eyes while addressing clients, board meetings or attending events.

I went into a period (heavy periods or non-existent, the Russian roulette of menstrual cycles, but I digress) of denial.

I just ignored it until inexplicably, the coup demanded more recognition, so as subtle as a marauding tank, brain fog, scarcity of sleep, hair/skin issues, more hot sweats, and pain invaded.

I found the psychological warfare darkly fascinating; I can only verbalise it this way: it seemed to whisper in a thick hypnotic Russian accent, "Darlink' you know you can't do this" at the most inopportune moments. Her way of speaking reeked of concern and friendliness, but with an icy blade that she would happily run through my heart, all still with a smile on her face and perfectly manicured hands.

'Olga' spread self-doubt and anxiety through my veins like only poisonous propaganda can. I was fortunate that I could use techniques to combat this influx due to my university training and years of work experience; however, sometimes her dulcet, persuasive tones would permeate, leaving me feeling exposed and anxious.

My period of denial and my menstrual cycle came to a halt two years after that first hot flush. I was relieved that my periods had stopped; I flashed back to a memory where I came home from school at age 13 with a wad of toilet paper in my knickers, as I had started bleeding in chemistry (ironically, in the 'first period' as we referred to our lessons) I wailed to my mum "What? I have to endure this every month?" Then dissolved into gut-wrenching sobs.

For many women, the biological clock and the ending of periods is an immense source of sorrow and devastation.

Hot Mess Self-Help

The night sweats became another semantic field of war, as it turned to rely on hand-to-hand combat using flame throwers to ignite my very flesh. I would be left with an outline of my body imprinted on the sheets in a hot liquid glaze.

I began to seek help and support through literature and social media. I quickly sifted through the: You can look as good as me; I discovered the secret to menopause; I have done a 3-hour course online; so now I am a Meno coach or I flew through meno-subtext (as I am so much better than you) type groups/sites.

I filed these under, 'Bit patronising but bravo for seeing the market potential.' However, clients brought to my attention their feelings that these types of 'Support' can feel very punishing to women who are barely hanging on raising children, keeping a career or roof over their head, looking after ageing parents and trying to keep a relationship together, whilst wading through fatigue, weight gain and mood swings.

I see through my work that although there is greater awareness, there is also a growing culture of blame and shame towards older women or women of any age suffering debilitating physical or emotional symptoms of menopause.

The flag of judgment should not be waved so readily as we go through this milestone in our lives. I also discovered some very interesting articles and books that have resonated with me, and spoken to some truly inspiring women in my search for answers to alleviate my symptoms.

The message was clear that we should all take responsibility for a balanced diet, exercise and self-care, but do not use this as a weapon against the sisterhood that has to work, has limited finances and has little downtime.

Personally speaking and through the experiences of many women I have worked with on a psychological basis, what I and they needed was empathy, candid sharing of experiences and certifiable options.

Once I discovered what I craved at this stage, I challenged myself to leave the internal battleground, not to accept my lot; I integrated elements of my training as a counsellor with the natural world and the female life cycle. To have survived the phases of maiden and mother and reached the crone stage is an honour.

I cherished my age, a richly deep and awakening part of our lives. We are wise ladies who have experiences and stories to share. The crone is no silver-haired, sweet old lady; she can embody chaos, shaking the foundations of what you have always done or roles placed upon us and showing that a new way of thinking and being is ready to emerge.

I began looking at MY needs; why was I suffering with a growing list of ailments? Why did I feel I had to cope?

I took stock and became my own best friend. I valued myself for being me; this was a challenging task and is still a work in progress. I threw aside the notion that if I asked for medical support, I had somehow failed. I called the GP and, after tests and consultations, began HRT.

It's early days; I am only a few months in, but the night sweats, joint pain and fatigue have gone. I am sleeping more and looking at what I want to achieve in these glorious but challenging days of reflection; now, I am not so besieged by my imagined war of menopause.

Olga is no match for the crone…

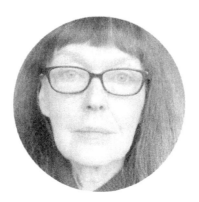

ANDREA HOCHGATTERER

AFTER A TWENTY-YEAR CAREER IN THE FILM AND ENTERTAINMENT INDUSTRY, AUSTRIAN-BORN ANDREA FOLLOWED HER PASSION FOR NATURAL HEALING AND RETRAINED AS A CAM PRACTITIONER. SHE NOW SUPPORTS CLIENTS ALL OVER THE WORLD WITH HER UNIQUE 1-2-1 MINDBODYALIGNMENT PROGRAMMES.

EXPLORING WRITING AS A WAY TO REGAIN HER INNER VOICE, ANDREA HAS WRITTEN VARIOUS ARTICLES AND CONTRIBUTED TO COLLABORATIVE BOOKS BEFORE BRANCHING OUT AS THE LEAD AUTHOR AND CREATOR OF "THE STRESS MAZE". AFTER WINNING THE NANOWRIMO WRITING COMPETITION THROUGH THE BOOK CHIEF PUBLISHING HOUSE, SHE IS NOW WRITING HER DEBUT NOVEL.

MINDBODYALIGNMENT.CO.UK
HOCHGATTERERA@AOL.COM

Chapter 2

BEYOND BIOLOGY, MY WALK TO FREEDOM.

By Andrea Hochgatterer

Menopause is a total misnomer as far as I am concerned because menstruation does not just pause; it reduces its frequency and then stops.

Or is it meant to tell us to pause mid-life?

Now, that would be more along my line of thinking.

I prefer to call it 'The Change' because this is exactly how I experienced it.

On the surface, we are simply changing from one hormonal state into another, and whilst many have no problem understanding their hormones, there is more to it.

I found acceptance of what was happening and staying curious about the changes, even when at times I reminded myself of my teenage self, grumpily swinging through my moods.

These were major components for staying sane throughout the process.

I was relieved when I hit menopause; compared to my periods, it seemed like a dawdle.

After the first moment of hick-up as I had not understood instantly what was happening, five years into a new relationship and settling down with my new partner, at the age of forty-three, I had started missing periods. There was no chance of me being pregnant as my partner had had a vasectomy; my body clearly understood it was time to start slowly withdrawing from this part of my journey.

There is no possibility of kids, so why bother?

And boy, was I glad.

I had suffered from the beginning of my periods with twenty-one-day cycles and bleeds lasting up to seven days and heavy to boot, flushing and gushing all over the place, like the tap that could not be shut off.

I remember in my teenage years, when sanitary products weren't exactly high-tech, I more than once jumped out of a cab coming back from a party, jumping terrified, as I could feel the blood soaking through my trousers, jumping in the hope I had not leaked onto the cab seat; oh the embarrassment of it!

My cycles had a significant impact on my general energy levels, and topping this, I was constantly cold and had terrible circulation.

They said it was iron deficiency, or as I would come to understand, a permanent state of stress and freeze response. I won't go into this as it would make for a wholly different article.

I love the idea in Eastern philosophy that menopause can be compared to the Kundalini rising experience.

The power rising within ourselves to connect to self and a higher state of being in increased consciousness, where we don't identify ourselves as females only. Walking the earth fulfilling our duties via oestrogen and progesterone-driven mechanisms to ensure the survival of the species, instead stepping into a new energy of being us.

Anyway, back to my story.

All that lost energy, the state of freeze, the prison of living with periods (they used to call it the curse, I do understand) suddenly, the onset of peri-menopause changed me into a state of high energy, creativity was no longer pumped into releasing blood from my womb. Instead, like a veil lifting, I suddenly had the energy, the inspiration and the will to take my life in a different direction.

In a way, I counted myself lucky despite hot flushes, which were welcome. I loved the fact that I wasn't cold any longer, perfect circulation, hot hands and most of all, cosy warm feet in bed at night. One jumper instead of five!

Sweating out toxins at night is great; there is no need for a sauna.

Three t-shirts lined up at the foot end of the bed, to change soaked ones into dry, back to sleep I went, cosy and warm.

So scarce and scant periods, warm body, full of creativity… I hit the ground running.

I started studying again, first Naturopathic Nutrition, then Craniosacral Therapy, which helped me immensely to put the right things into place to experience a smoother transition.

My go-to support for physical, mental and emotional support were:

consuming food full of phyto oestrogen,

adaptogenic herbs as supplements and tinctures,

weight-bearing exercise

meditation,

transdermal creams; at first, wild Yam and later natural identical hormones.

A new purpose and massive goal I was ready to achieve.

The most amazing experience was stepping out of the box of being a female and conforming to society's demands.

All the uncertainties about a woman's role shifted, and I became just me.

My thinking changed; I could now choose how and what I wanted to be, and worries about how the world experienced me had become unimportant.

Before I conclude this article, I must mention an observation about menopause…

I had my last period, age fifty-two, and thought I was on the home straight feeling brilliant, which I did for five years; however, after suffering a series of major bereavements that took over my life, I had to re-evaluate.

The signs and symptoms of grief were similar to what women can experience during menopause, and the line for me was indistinguishable.

Extreme tiredness, brain fog, short memory span, a lacklustre existence.

I feel it is worth mentioning for the readers' benefit that, going through menopause, many women are confronted with other life-changing experiences like bereavement, caring for ageing parents, and suffering empty nest syndrome, all of which contribute to stress in our daily lives, impacting our hormones and creating a less smooth ride through menopause.

The Change, like the teenage years, is a transition from one form of being human to another, a step into a different kind of being where we finally can experience ourselves at the core of our being.

We are becoming not less but more than just a woman; we have the chance to get to know ourselves all over again, see ourselves in a different light, donning different spectacles and seeing the world through a different lens.

The lens of that of a human being goes beyond biology.

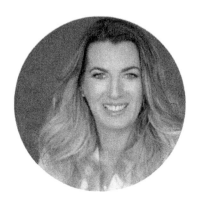

CAT ROBINSON ARMOR

CAT ROBINSON ARMOR, AKA THE HORMONE FAIRY, IS A CERTIFIED MENOPAUSE HEALTH COACH, AN EXPERIENCED HOMEOPATH WITH TRAINING IN NUTRITION AND HERBS, A HYPNOTHERAPIST AND A DUTCH TEST EXPERT.

CAT'S EXPERIENCE IN THESE ALTERNATIVE THERAPIES ALLOWS HER TO GIVE YOU A HOLISTIC APPROACH TO PERI-MENOPAUSE AND POST-MENOPAUSE THAT A DOCTOR CAN'T.

FOR YEARS, HER PASSION HAS BEEN WORKING WITH WOMEN LIKE YOU WHO STRUGGLE WITH MENOPAUSAL SYMPTOMS OR WHO MAY FEEL FRUSTRATED WITH THE MEDICAL PROFESSION. HER SKILLS AND TRAINING MEAN SHE IS UNIQUELY PLACED TO GUIDE YOU ON HOW TO SURVIVE THE MENOPAUSE TRANSITION NATURALLY OR ALONGSIDE MEDICATION.

WWW.THEHORMONEFAIRY.CO.UK
INFO@THEHORMONEFAIRY.CO.UK

Chapter 3

RELIEF OR RUIN, HRT'S NIGHTMARE

By Cat Robinson Armor

Hormone Replacement Therapy (HRT) can be the wonder drug providing instant relief for many women going through perimenopause, but there isn't a one-size-fits-all, and for some, HRT can be the start of the nightmare and menopause hell.

Progesterone made Jayne feel suicidal.

Jayne found me when I presented "The Upgrade Menopause & Mental Health" Lunch & Learn session at her company.

I'd mentioned that women who experienced hormonal depression in the past, during puberty, alongside their monthly menstrual cycle or post-natal, were more likely to experience it again in the perimenopause.

Jayne had depression in her early 20's when she took the birth control pill. Now at 47, with fluctuating periods and low moods, she was prescribed oestrogen gel and progesterone tablets.

Two weeks of the month were absolute hell for her. Her mood plummeted as soon as she started the 14-day progesterone cycle. She didn't want to get out of bed, took long-term sick leave from her career, and didn't see the point in life despite having two wonderful children.

In complete desperation, Jayne picked up the phone and called me. Thankfully, I was in between clients and had time to listen. My motto is, "Menopause does not have to be miserable; no one should be held hostage to their hormones". I assured Jayne that she had not gone crazy and that it sounded like she could be progesterone intolerant. This is when you are sensitive to the hormone, usually in its synthetic form, such as progestogen, and symptoms can be like premenstrual syndrome or Premenstrual dysphoric disorder (PMDD).

Progesterone medication is needed alongside oestrogen replacement for women with a uterus, usually for a minimum of 12 days a month. This is to prevent the endometrium from becoming too thick and minimise the risk of cells in the lining turning cancerous. For most women, progesterone makes us feel great; it's the calming hormone - for others like Jayne, it can make you feel awful, emotional, or even suicidal.

I advised Jayne to speak with her GP as to other options, such as changing the dose of the progesterone or the number of days or to try other forms of progesterone, such as the Mirena coil or local progesterone (a tablet inserted into the vagina at night).

Alternatively, I could help her with natural remedies to help the mood swings, adding herbs and nutrition to boost her levels.

When it comes to herbal tinctures, it's essential to research or speak to a qualified practitioner - especially if you are on medication, as some herbal medicines and tinctures can have a negative response.

After a discussion with her GP, Jayne chose to take a short break from the HRT medication, adding the recommended herbs and supplements to increase her levels naturally.

Here are a few of the remedies Jayne added:

- Chasteberry or vitex agnus-castus, as it's often known, is a herb known to decrease prolactin levels, which helps balance oestrogen and progesterone.

This can be a useful remedy for women in early perimenopause, as it can increase the release of luteinising hormone (LH); closer to menopause, women lose the ovarian response to the herb.

- Vitamin C, A, E, B6, Zinc and fatty acids to help.
- Seed cycling with sunflower and sesame seeds.

Within a few months, Jayne was back in control of her emotions and able to return to work.

Oestrogen was causing Donna's misery!

As soon as Donna turned 40, she started to experience a lack of motivation, absolutely no desire for sex, as well as low energy and cravings in the afternoon. Her waistband and thighs began to increase; she felt "urgh".

After watching a documentary on TV, she figured out it must be perimenopause and took herself off to her GP. Without many questions, Donna walked out with a prescription for oestrogen patches, progesterone tablets and testosterone gel. She thought she was doing the right thing; the documentary said going on HRT early was beneficial!

Donna was a little scared to try the testosterone gel, so leaving that in her bedside drawer, she started with the oestrogen patches and progesterone pills. It wasn't the wonder drug she had hoped for - her weight continued to increase, she was now experiencing headaches, and her period cycle went from a regular 28-day to every three weeks with spotting and 10-day bleeds.

In her follow-up phone consultation, the GP changed the prescription to oestrogen gel, increasing the dose, not something she felt comfortable with.

Donna came for a DUTCH Test (Dried Urine Test for Comprehensive Hormones) and a consultation with me to check her levels and to see how she could improve her symptoms. It's a simple urine test taken at home that looks at your primary sex hormones, oestrogen metabolites, cortisol, DHEA & androgens, and nutritional markers.

Her DUTCH test results showed oestrogen dominance. All her primary oestrogens, oestrone, Oestradiol and oestriol, were high; more importantly, the oestrogen detoxification was poor.

Whilst oestrogen is beneficial, we must use and lose it, detoxing it out of the system. Otherwise, oestrogen can stay in the bloodstream, leading to oestrogen-dominant symptoms, PMS, water retention, migraines, and heavy periods, putting you at greater risk of developing oestrogen-linked cancers. All new symptoms Donna has been experiencing since starting the HRT.

Testosterone was in the low range; that hormone can be linked to your mojo, motivation and libido. It does decrease with age, and sometimes testosterone can convert into oestradiol, causing oestrogen to rise.

Finally, dopamine, the pleasure-seeking hormone, was low, hence her cravings for sugar, carbs and alcohol later in the day.

Donna focused on her liver health to detox the oestrogen, adding DIM, a supplement, to support this. The testosterone gel was a good option for Donna; she could add Zinc, Maca root and more weight-bearing exercises to boost levels.

With simple diet and lifestyle changes, Donna has increased her energy and found her zest for life.

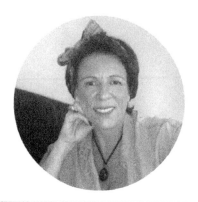

CHRISTINE WRIGHT

CHRISTINE WRIGHT IS A FORMER FUNCTIONING ALCOHOLIC, WHO IS NOW AN INSPIRING SPEAKER, (NOMINATED FOR INSPIRATIONAL WOMAN OF THE YEAR 2021), AUTHOR, MENTOR, BEHAVIOURAL CHANGE EXPERT, LIFESTYLE CHANGE EXPERT, FOUNDER OF SOCIAL SOBRIETY SOCIETY, FOUNDER OF HABIT BREAKER - A MOTIVATIONAL COMMUNITY THAT EMPOWERS WOMEN AND TEENAGE GIRLS.
IT WAS A DIVINE INTERVENTION THAT TOOK PLACE IN 2019 WHICH LED HER TO CHANGE HER DESTRUCTIVE CYCLE AND PATTERN OF BEHAVIOURS, WHICH HAD GOVERNED HER LIFE SINCE BEING 14 YEARS OLD AND HELPED HER CARVE OUT A HEALTHIER PATH IN MIND, BODY, AND SOUL OF WHICH SHE NOW SHARES HER UNIQUE REFRAMING METHOD.WITH WOMEN AND TEENAGE GIRLS.

HTTPS://LINKTR.EE/HABITBREAKER

Chapter 4

FEELING LESS PORN STAR & MORE MENOPAUSAL MONSTER?

By Christine Wright

OK, let's not beat around the bush!

I'm keeping this real; I am not speaking of huge pert breasts bouncing up and down with nipples so erect that they look like they have had ice cubes rubbed all over them or moist vaginas (yes, I am going there). It's more of a breasts like spaniels ears, and dry vaginas party that's just welcomed you into the club, right?

How very rude? What gives me the right to comment so crudely?

Well, here's the scoop; I'm Chrissie, a former functioning alcoholic who is peri-menopausal, and I have an online habit-breaking community, where most of my gorgeous ladies trust me to mentor them through their unhealthy drinking habits.

We tend to find that through our workings together, we often speak of 'menopausal chaos' and how fuelling that chaos with alcohol is most definitely going to make you hot as hell and not in a pre-mentioned porn star way, more of a dishevelled Patsy way from the great British comedy, Absolutely Fabulous.

So why do we consume alcohol whilst going through this chaos? Why do we think we can become the greatest mixologist in life and keep everything afloat like those three coffee beans you get atop your espresso martini?

Truth bomb – We can't; menopause is a natural phase in a woman's life that marks the end of her reproductive years. This brings many physical and emotional changes that can vary from woman to woman. During this time, it is essential to prioritise self-care, make positive choices and maybe implement new holistic habits to nurture our overall well-being, including our relationship with alcohol.

So, before we go any further, I need to ask you a few questions and be honest; otherwise, those nipples of yours will soon be touching your knees. Forget Pinocchio's nose; it's all about nipple action and defying gravity.

"What is your relationship with alcohol – good, bad, not sure?"

"What are your Whys? Why do you feel the need to drink daily, drink socially, binge drink?"

"How does it make you feel - When drinking it, having drunk it, the next morning?"

"Have the effects of drinking changed through your journey of menopause?"

You must understand the reasonings behind these questions and your relationship with alcohol and get to grips with the implications of how detrimental it can be both short-term and long-term on your health, including mind, body and soul, more so, through your menopausal chaos cycle.

In this chapter, we will explore and list the effects of alcohol on menopause and discuss strategies for maintaining a balanced and healthy lifestyle and finding you again. This is addressed in much more detail and tailored to individuals when we go through the REFRAMING methodology at Habit Breaker.

This does not mean we become boring, less fun, less wild because we have limited or no party juice.

Effects of Alcohol on Menopause

1. Hormonal Imbalance: You're all over the place right now, and any alcohol consumption can disrupt the delicate hormonal balance already affected by menopause.

Regular drinking can interfere with the production and regulation of hormones, potentially exacerbating symptoms such as hot flushes and mood swings.

2. Sleep Disruption: Menopause often brings about difficulties in sleeping, and alcohol can further disrupt sleep patterns.

While it may initially help you fall asleep faster, alcohol can lead to fragmented and poor-quality sleep, leaving you feeling groggy and fatigued the next day.

3. Increased Hot Flushes: Hot flushes and night sweats are common menopausal symptoms that can be intensified by alcohol consumption.

Alcohol acts as a vasodilator, expanding blood vessels and triggering hot flushes. It can also worsen the severity and frequency of these episodes, causing discomfort and distress.

4. Bone Health: Menopause is associated with a decline in bone density, increasing the risk of osteoporosis. Alcohol, especially when consumed excessively, can further weaken bones and contribute to the developing of this condition. It is crucial to be mindful of our alcohol intake and prioritise bone-strengthening activities like regular exercise and a balanced diet.

So how the 'frickety frack' do we navigate all these shenanigans whilst cutting back or cutting out alcohol completely?

Well, we REFRAME our relationship with the bottle. It is advisable to moderate alcohol consumption during menopause; it does not necessarily mean complete abstinence.

However, most of my lovely ladies develop a new zest for life and alcohol just is not included and given the time of day anymore. That time is now spent on self-love, self-acceptance, setting boundaries and developing new, healthier habits.

Below, I've listed some helpful strategies to maintain a balanced and healthy lifestyle during this menopause hell phase for you:

1. Educate Yourself: Understanding your relationship between alcohol and menopause. This is the first step towards making informed decisions. Hence why, I set you the questions above. You need to have an honest approach to your drinking habits and why they present themselves.

If you find alcohol problematic, find communities online or in person, health professionals, and mentors who can help you gain a healthier approach to alcohol and keep you accountable.

2. Moderation is Key: If you choose to consume alcohol, do so in moderation. The Alcohol guidelines state that women should not exceed 14 units per week, and it is advisable to spread your drinking over three days or more. (UK Chief Medical Officers Low-Risk Drinking Guidelines)

To give some substance, 14 units equate to 6 glasses of wine (175ml 13%ABV), 14 single measures of spirit (25ml 40%ABV) or 6 Pints of ordinary strength beer/cider/lager (68ml 4%ABV) (Alcohol Change UK)

It is important to note that these guidelines may not be suitable for everyone, particularly those with certain medical conditions or who are taking specific medications. Consult your healthcare provider for personalised recommendations.

3. Alternative Coping Mechanisms: Instead of relying solely on alcohol to cope with menopausal symptoms, explore alternative strategies to manage stress and improve well-being. Engage in yoga, meditation, dance, deep breathing exercises, or mindfulness practices. Prioritise self-care and find healthy outlets for relaxation and emotional support.

4. Stay Hydrated and Nourished: Menopause can sometimes lead to dehydration, and alcohol can further exacerbate this issue. Ensure you stay adequately hydrated by drinking plenty of water and consuming hydrating foods like fruits and vegetables. Additionally, a balanced diet rich in nutrients can support overall health during menopause.

So let's wrap things up. Navigating menopause can be a unique and transformative journey for every woman.

By understanding the effects of alcohol on menopause and developing new healthier habits inclusive of holistic approaches to wellness, we can make informed choices that prioritise our physical and emotional well-being.

Remember, this chapter serves as a guide to help you make informed decisions, but it is always important to consult healthcare professionals for personalised advice tailored to your specific needs. As I am the queen of gratitude, even when the shit hits the fan (I always find the lesson in that, so I don't rinse and repeat), I ask you to embrace this phase of life the best you can with grace, self-compassion, and a commitment to nurturing your overall health and remember you are a star. Be it an alter ego porn star or a twinkly star, I will let you choose but know this you will soon shine bright again as this phase will soon pass.

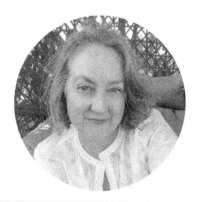

ELLE BRIGHT

ELLE IS A SCIENTIST, ARTIST, AUTHOR AND SPEAKER WHO SPECIALISES IN MINDSET FOR WOMEN ENTREPRENEURS SCALING THEIR BUSINESS TO 7-FIGURES AND BEYOND TO MAKE QUANTUM LEAPS – THE BIG SHIFTS THAT ALLOW YOU TO EARN MORE, WORK LESS, AND ENJOY IT ALL – SO THAT YOU CAN BE THE WOMEN WHO CREATES AND CATALYSES THE CHANGE YOU WANT TO SEE IN THE WORLD.

AS A MINDSET COACH, HYPNOTHERAPIST AND MIND-BODY CONNECTION EXPERT, SHE SUPPORTS YOU WITH HIGH-PERFORMANCE NEUROSCIENCE TO RELEASE, OVERCOME AND TRANSFORM THE LIMITING BELIEFS THAT CAUSE BURNOUT AND RELATIONSHIP DAMAGE AND CREATE YOUR CUSTOM LIFE-WORK HARMONY WITHOUT SACRIFICE.

ELLEBRIGHT.COM
ELLEBRIGHT@ELLEBRIGHT.CO.UK

Chapter 5

MENOPAUSE, WOMEN AND WHALES

By Elle Bright

Did you know that humans are the only mammal species on the planet, along with all toothed whales – belugas, narwhals, short-finned pilot whales and orcas – that experience menopause?

Menopause is an evolutionary mystery. It prima facie runs contrary to Darwinian natural selection, which prioritises reproduction. We should reproduce until we die. And most women did until advances in health meant that we began to outlive our reproductive window.

Data for Europe and North America give an age of about 51 for menopause, so most women born before 1880 never experienced life after menopause. In the 1880s, life expectancy was just 29 years. With improvements in health, this reached 42 for women by 1900, and in North America and Western Europe, it rocketed up to 68 in 1950. Now it's 82, and we know that a girl born in 2020 has a life expectancy of 90.

So, it's only in recent history that most women are significantly outliving our reproductive window. Our lifespan will include over

30 years beyond menopause, making up more than one-third of our lives.

In fact, until a few generations ago, this led the Western medical system to consider menopause to be a deficiency disease.

In the Victorian period, leeching, cold baths and sedatives were prescribed, and hygiene and "moral management" was emphasised. In the 1930s, therapies included animals' crushed ovaries and testicular juice. The primary ingredient of one of the first oestrogen pills, introduced in 1942, was pregnant-mare urine!

Since then, there have been a number of serious side effects with synthetic oestrogen, and even today, Hormone Replacement Therapy (HRT) is known to be related to potentially life-threatening blood clots and may increase the risk of breast cancer and dementia. Yet heart disease, osteoporosis, and Alzheimer's disease are all known to be linked to the lower oestrogen levels of perimenopausal and menopausal women. We do not yet know enough about the long-term safety of HRT, and we need to. Fast.

The transition around menopause (12 months after the last menstrual cycle) can last up to 20 years; the female body takes eight to ten years in preparation for menopause (perimenopause) and can experience menopausal symptoms ten years after the occurrence of menopause (post-menopause). The number of menopausal women worldwide is estimated to reach 1.1 billion by 2025.

In 2020, the Female Founders Fund survey reported that 78% of women said that menopause had interfered with their lives, but Bonafide Health indicated in 2021 that 73% of women who were experiencing "symptoms" weren't seeking treatment and that societal stigma was the primary cause.

The North American Menopause Society has found that a woman has twice the chance of developing depression during this time. Mental health issues, of course, are exacerbated by the varied physical, mental, and emotional symptoms of the transition.

This is in stark contrast to non-Western cultures, which see menopause as a beautiful and even celebratory time of change and freedom.

Interestingly, research shows that menopausal "symptoms" are not universal but appear strongly influenced by the cultural environment. Cultures celebrating menopause or which more positively view women's ageing and menopause, experience fewer unpleasant effects.

I understand all this to mean that menopausal "symptoms" are a worldwide issue, and we need to change the narrative from the stigma of ageing to the celebration of the witch, hag, goddess and crone. This archetype embodies women's instinctive ways of channelling wisdom, inner knowing, and intuition that honours older women. Crone comes from the crown; hag comes from hagio, meaning holy; and witch comes from wit, meaning wise. It is time to reclaim the power of the third age of womanhood. The first being girlhood, the second as womanhood and the third and final as the time of wise womanhood.

I advocate that every woman needs to stand up for her health and the health of all women by speaking up and dispelling the stigma. As a mindset expert, I know this isn't easy to do, but here is some general guidance on what any woman can do.

First, you can keep a diary and note down details about anything you are experiencing that is negatively affecting your life that could be a "symptom". Second, you can be proactive and do all you can to look after your health with nutrition, hydration, sleep, moving your body and fresh air to reduce those factors.

Third, you can participate in communities promoting women's menopausal awareness and health. And, when you discuss your health with your health professional, do so with the confidence and conviction that you know your body better than anyone else can and stay the course (change professionals if you need to), get the help you need for your health concerns and tell other women about it – not as medical advice but as information because every woman who speaks up helps all women.

So ... why do toothed whales outlive menopause, too? They don't have healthcare systems to extend their lifespan that we do. There are theories on why a species would need a reason to stop reproducing and live on afterwards. As highly intelligent and social creatures, orca research shows they are matriarchal. Orcas live in family pods where both male and female offspring stay with their mother for their entire lives. The oldest female, the matriarch, leads the pod to their hunting grounds, and offspring are raised with the help of other females in the pod. Did you know that several human matriarchies exist today (but not a lot of data as to their menopausal experience) and that it has been postulated that all of humankind was a matriarch in the past? So maybe outliving menopause is evolutionary after all.

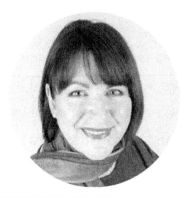

ELLIE LACROSSE

ELLIE IS A PUBLISHED AUTHOR, WRITER, AWARD
WINNING POET AND OWNER OF A SMALL WRITING
RETREAT, 'HEARTEN HOUSE' IN CUMBRIA, UK.

HER CAREER HAS SPANNED SEVERAL DECADES
IN THE CONSTRUCTION INDUSTRY, TEACHING
AND RETRAINING AS A REFLEXOLOGIST. SHE HAS
A PROPERTY PORTFOLIO AND RUNS HER OWN
AIRBNB HOLIDAY LETS.

ELLIE IS NOW LIVING A MORE CREATIVE
LIFESTYLE AND LOVES SUPPORTING THE
CREATIVITY OF OTHER WOMEN.

ELLIE@LITTLEREDTYPERITER.COM

Chapter 6

TESTIMONY OF FECUNDITY

By Ellie LaCrosse

My fertility died a long, slow, painful, complex death over my most productive fertile years. For about fifteen years, I had 'issues' resulting in my own 'Menopause Hell'.

I shall recount my personal story, hoping that other younger women will have the confidence to insist on investigations through their GP's and recognise signs and symptoms within themselves or with their partners.

With no disrespect to the many authors who are therapists, there came a time when no about of pain management techniques, CBT, clearing my chakras, drinking green juices and singing 'Kumbaya' made a jot of difference to the pain I experienced.

Endometriosis is a condition where skin tissue similar to the lining of the womb wall grows into other organs or tissue, such as the uterus, ovaries, fallopian tubes or within the body cavity, sticking to the bowel or other organs.

It swells and contracts over the monthly cycle, and the pain associated with this condition can and has led some women to suicide; such is the excruciatingly debilitating nature of the waves of pain that can be experienced. It is often misdiagnosed as other conditions like IBS or chronic back/pelvic pain, fatigue and depression or early menopause symptoms.

It impacted my pain levels during my periods, sexual intercourse, and bowel movements. It ruined an earlier serious relationship and affected my teaching career because I had so much time off work. It took seven years to finally get my first diagnosis, my first keyhole surgery to scrape endometrial material off organs and inside my womb. The first couple of years were better. I still had very painful periods, but it was a couple of days of intense pain that I generally could cope with.

In addition, my husband was still working for a major Corporation. As part of his salary package, we enjoyed free healthcare. I was entitled to wife benefits, and the company arranged for me to have private surgery, which I was incredibly grateful for.

Another seven or eight years passed, and my monthly cycle became more erratic and painful until I reached my breaking point. I was in my early fifties, thinking I was becoming 'menopausal' with the occasional tsunami of drenching hot sweats.

I spent so much time in pain, resting in bed for half of each month; life seemed too painful to continue living. To my shame, I genuinely considered suicide.

Although my long-suffering husband was very supportive, our sex life had dropped off the cliff. He was working out his notice to take early retirement from work. He was looking forward to doing more things together with me and travelling. I felt like a fraud as far as being a wife to him. One day, alone in our home in extreme pain, I reached for the whisky bottle to try to blot out everything. It didn't work; I became nauseous and unsteady, tripping over and gashing my hand badly as I went to the bathroom.

As I sat on the floor, blood smeared on the tiles, I started to howl in pain and disgust at myself. I hauled myself up, flung open the bathroom cabinet and made a pill mountain on the floor. I distinctly remember saying to myself, "If I'm going to do this, I'd better do it right; I don't want to wake up".

Suddenly, I heard my husband's voice downstairs; he'd come home earlier from work. He came bounding up the stairs and stood in horror at the scene before him. He scooped me up and held me very tightly. He'd put two and two together rapidly and burst into tears,

"Ellie, no, no, no! There's got to be something to help you!"

When I cried out, he helped me to the bedroom to rest. He said I needed to talk to someone and return to my GP.

"Oh yeah? The same GP that said only last week that I was having symptoms because I was a 'little bit fat'? The bitch! I asked for a hysterectomy, and what did she say to me, remember? 'You're looking at a waiting list of at least two years on the NHS. I suggest you have CBT and lose a couple of stones!'"

"Ellie, you need to talk to someone and look into having a Hysterectomy privately."

So, later that evening, I phoned the charity' Endometriosis UK' helpline. Two hours later, chatting to an anonymous but empathetic volunteer gave me some contact details of a well-qualified Endocrinologist working out of a private hospital near Manchester.

I did have a Hysterectomy operation privately a few weeks later. It cost £11,000 (all of my savings at the time and some on the credit card) because of complications during surgery. However, after the healing period, I finally had a pain-free life back, only to face another dilemma a few years later.

No one had mentioned that I needed to top up my depleted Oestrogen hormones and that I'd immediately feel the full effects of menopause.

I believe we women still have to fight for some basic aid to the natural transitions we will all face as we age. I also feel like I'm the generation that missed the opening up of this once-taboo subject. I've never had conversations with the womenfolk in my family about menopause, or at best, limited conversations from my mother, who, in an act of martyrdom, precedes every conversation with "We just got on with it".

I give back to the charity Endometriosis UK whenever I can. Their kindness and empathy saved my life.

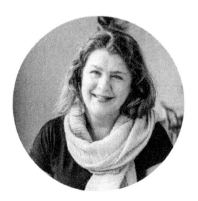

FEMKE WILLIAMS

FEMKE WILLIAMS IS A DUTCH-BORN FORMER NURSE WHO'S BEEN IN THE UK SINCE 1999.

FEMKE IS NOW, BASED AT HOME IN WORKSOP AND WORKS AS A WELLBEING AND SOUL COACH AND MENTOR, INTEGRATING NATURAL THERAPIES, FATIGUE RECOVERY SPECIALISM AND THE HEALING ARTS (MUSIC, MOVEMENT/EMBODIMENT & ART) INTO HER SERVICES.

FEMKE HAS A SPECIAL INTEREST IN BURNOUT PREVENTION AND RECOVERY FOR HEALTH PROFESSIONALS AND HELPS OTHERS CULTIVATE SELF-CARE, SELF-LOVE, COURAGE & CONFIDENCE TO CREATE A LIFE THEY LOVE!

ROSEWOODWELLBEING.CO.UK
FEMKE@ROSEWOODWELLBEING.CO.UK

Chapter 7

MOVING THROUGH, NATURALLY

By Femke Williams

I have been called a 'Witch' because I describe myself as a 'healer' and feel that I resonate with the spiritual tradition of self-exploration and self-awareness. I am honoured! Because the essence of witchcraft lies in the philosophy of life, in the meaning *behind* the rituals, the texts, and the full moon celebrations.

Being a Witch is not about calling out the incantations, having altars at home and brewing herbal drinks (although I am sure some find that fun). What makes a woman a Witch is her willingness to broaden her consciousness and awareness.

Looking for knowledge requires action. There are no written theories in a holy book, but I can find this knowledge within Nature, within myself and others. I am looking for the knowledge of experienced, 'lived through' wisdom.

A Witch would never lock herself up with one way of thinking and deny all other opinions and ways of thinking. Because then, her development would be one-sided and eventually stagnate.

No, she must open her heart and mind to different cultures, traditions and beliefs compared to herself.

In the 'old religion', women after their 50th birthday were seen as the old wise ones; 50 is a 'crone' year, or the year after menopause (for most women now between 45-55).

But, in our society, she has become almost invisible. She doesn't speak up because she has learned not to assert herself. She doesn't feel she can contribute anything meaningful because nobody asks her what she thinks and feels. Although it's getting more attention now because menopause is much more talked about in the media, she is still virtually non-existent!

Her world, her vision and her experience do not get much attention; if she is at all portrayed in a TV series or film, she is reduced to a sexless, visionless grandma who, at most, deserves a smile.

But deep down, you and I know that we will always have something to give that can help a younger generation, even if they don't know it (yet).

Having spent years working in Health, Wellbeing and Energy medicine, I have deepened my knowledge about the entangled workings of the body, mind, spirit & soul. So, how can we best help ourselves and other women move through the stages of menopause naturally? To have fewer or less severe symptoms, more ease and understanding, and create more self-love?

I am aware that many women now enter the stages of pre- and perimenopause earlier (i.e. induced after hysterectomy or hormonal imbalances due to other causes) OR later (as we are living longer) than before.

For a good year now (since turning 48), I have been experiencing hot flashes, brain fog, indigestion, irritability and recently, I have noticed my blood pressure is too high. A sore and slightly swollen left ankle most days and exploding periods irregularly with 2 or 3 months in between.

I have recently been to the GP to have my blood pressure, bloods, and heart checked; my symptoms are hormonal and can be addressed to a certain extent with lifestyle changes and a natural diet. Still, it needs checking medically to rule out any underlying conditions causing this symptom. Other symptoms (increased headaches, irritability) do not interfere with my daily activities and happiness level as I find ways to attend to my needs (i.e. rest, meditate).

However, what I see happening, due to research and available information to us all via the internet, whether true or false, is that most women come to a conclusion about their symptoms and why these exist and turn to the medical world for a quick-fix or magic pill to make them better. Now I am sure we'd all want rid of the symptoms of night sweats, brain fog, hot flashes, irritability, palpitations, painful & swollen joints, vaginal dryness and increasing migraines. However, to a certain extent, it is something that we have to acknowledge, accept and embrace. The body is changing, and we need to focus on giving it the best conditions to maintain the best possible health at these stages of transitioning.

Due to a drop in female hormones during the menopausal stages, some physical symptoms will be the same for many.

The key to experiencing less severe symptoms is to look at key areas in our lives that need addressing or that need our love and attention the most. Here, we see an unbreakable link to our emotional health, financial situation, movement, nutrition, environment, lifestyle & pace, relationships and Life Purpose (linked to spirituality). Together, these areas have a massive effect on our hormonal health, particularly the adrenal glands (negatively affected by stress of all kinds) and the thyroid gland (affected by trauma/stress/shock). It means that if we do not provide the correct environment, kindness and nourishment for our bodies, our immune system is compromised, and the body reacts with pain, auto-immunity, inflammation and disease. Put menopause on top of an already stressful life, with the hormonal balance being disrupted, which becomes a big ask for the body.

My conclusion is that we can do various things to help our body, mind, and soul prepare for this stage in our life. If we haven't done much of that before menopause start, it is never too late to support the body with kind thoughts, nutritious food, natural herbs, self-love (acceptance), relaxation therapies (e.g. reflexology, reiki) and positive attention (self-care).

I know it's much easier said than done, but we are in so much more control than we may believe, and we can let our 'Witchy Roots' help us to commit to our Well-being.

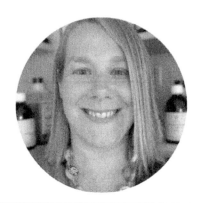

HANNAH CHARMAN

HANNAH HAS WORKED IN ALTERNATIVE MEDICINE SINCE SHE WAS 16 AND GRADUATED WITH A DEGREE IN WESTERN HERBAL MEDICINE IN 1999. SINCE THEN, SHE HAS RUN A THRIVING HERBAL PRACTICE AND TRAINED IN ADVANCED HYPNOTHERAPY AND IRIDOLOGY.

HANNAH FOUND HERSELF ENTERING PERIMENOPAUSE IN HER LATE 30'S, AND AFTER SEEING HOW EFFECTIVE HERBS WERE FOR HER, SHE SPECIALISED IN SUPPORTING WOMEN WITH HERBAL ALTERNATIVES TO HRT. SHE NOW COMBINES PRESCRIBED HERBAL TREATMENT WITH HEALTH COACHING AND/OR HYPNOTHERAPY TO HELP WOMEN REGAIN CONTROL ON EVERY LEVEL. HANNAH SEES PATIENTS ONLINE AND FROM HER CLINIC IN SHROPSHIRE.

PHYSICHEALTH.UK
HANNAH@PHYSICHEALTH.UK

Chapter 8

WHAT IF HRT ISN'T FOR ME?!

By Hannah Charman

Around 1/3 of women would prefer to get through menopause without HRT, either for medical reasons or because they prefer more natural approaches to most things. But for those with severe symptoms, not having access to the 'quick fix' that HRT can offer can make it all the more difficult.

I found myself beyond mainstream help with my health issues at 14. I was introduced to alternative medicine because it was the only option if I wanted to get better. For the most part, I've managed without mainstream healthcare ever since. Despite a history of serious menopausal mental illness in my family, I choose not to take HRT, preferring to use herbal medicines, good nutrition and lifestyle changes.

So, here's what I've found works as a peri-menopausal woman and a medical herbalist specialising in menopause. I hope it gives you some ideas too.

1 – Always Start with Self Care

The transition in menopause is a huge ask of the body. However, given the right resources, we can still do it fairly easily.

The problem is that we have put ourselves last for decades by the time we reach peri-menopause.

A chronically exhausted, stressed, and undernourished body will inevitably struggle to go through such a huge change, and it will complain as it does. So, see your symptoms as cries for help, and find little ways to support yourself through. Even small changes can make a huge difference not just in navigating menopause but way beyond too. For example, getting 30 minutes of exercise daily helps tame your hormones, manage your weight, and strengthen your bone, mental and heart health. It cuts your risk of dementia by a whopping 40%!

What small thing could you do today to take better care of yourself?

2 – Check in with Your Mind

Your mind plays various tricks on you throughout your life. It chatters away in the background, telling you you're not good enough, don't deserve to be happy, or can't do something you'd love to do. Now is a great time to listen to the chatter and watch your behaviour to see whether it's helping or holding you back.

A while ago, I realised that my joint pain, fatigue, and brain fog were possibly linked to a lack of exercise. The problem was that I had zero motivation to move despite knowing I'd soon feel much better if I could get more active.

I found a hypnotherapist to help me get motivated, and soon, I found myself in the swimming pool at 6.30 am several times a week. I loved it so much. I also found a swimming teacher to help me improve!

All my symptoms resolved within a couple of weeks, and every inch of me felt stronger, even my fingers!

If you feel you're holding yourself back in any way, hypnotherapy is a really quick way to replace those old patterns with more helpful ones. Alternatively, you could repeat positive affirmations like "I deserve to be happy and healthy" as you look in the mirror. It takes longer, but it doesn't cost a penny.

3 – Let Herbs Help!

Your ancestors would have used herbal medicines to fix every health issue, including menopause symptoms. Contrary to popular belief, menopause is not a new invention!

Suppose you were one of the lucky ones who survived multiple births, you'd probably have lived well beyond menopause. Nowadays, menopause is the only condition for which GPs are allowed to recommend herbs because there's plenty of evidence backing their use.

Prescribed herbal medicine gets incredible results when it comes to menopause symptoms. By prescribed herbal medicine, I mean taking a medicine that has been personalised to you following a consultation with a medical herbalist. Yes, it's an investment, but it saves all the wasted time and money trying to guess which herbal remedies to take, and it works fast, too!

Most of my patients see around an 80% improvement within 8-12 weeks, plus there's no weight gain or other side effects to worry about.

Many people don't realise that medical herbalists do more than prescribe herbs.

The health checks we do in the first consultation can help identify early warning signs of potential health problems. We can write to your GP to get some tests underway if you like. We also offer bucketfuls of moral support, advice, guidance and a good laugh at the end of a bad day.

Your medicine gets adjusted as you start to feel better, and we can work on other health issues at the same time as your menopause. We also keep you safe by checking that your herbs are safe to take alongside any other medication you're on. What's not to love?!

Pulling It All Together

We're complex beings, aren't we?! In my experience, if we want to get to the bottom of our health issues, we need to try and understand why they manifested in the first place. Whether we slap on a patch or take a pill or a herbal remedy, we miss the point if we don't listen to what our body is trying to tell us and act upon it. It might be that on a psycho-emotional level, we don't like ourselves much, so we stay up too late eating crisps on the sofa. In doing so, we deprive ourselves of restorative sleep and nourishing food. Our bodies then complain in the form of weight gain, anxiety, poor immunity, and crazy fluctuations in hormones. We know that we need to eat better, sleep more, and manage our stress, but if we subconsciously don't like ourselves, we won't find the motivation to do it. That's why it's OK to ask for and invest in some help, and if you can't do it now, when can you?

Hannah Charman is an experienced medical herbalist, health coach and advanced hypnotherapist offering natural health management for menopause. She works from her home in Shropshire and sees patients online too.

—

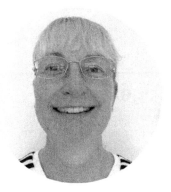

HELEN HELLIWELL

HELEN HELLIWELL IS THE OWNER OF BHB HEALTH AND FITNESS, IN HER 60'S AND POST-MENOPAUSE.

HER FACE-TO-FACE AND ONLINE BUSINESS FOCUSES ON COACHING LADIES OVER 40 TO THEIR VERY BEST HEALTH, WELLNESS, FITNESS AND GOAL ACHIEVEMENTS.

COMING FROM A WIDE VARIETY OF EMPLOYMENT, GETTING SUPER FIT AND STRONG AT 40 TO JOIN EMERGENCY SERVICES, ALONGSIDE RUNNING A HOUSE, WORKING, STUDYING AND THEN EXTENDING HER FAMILY AT 47, HELEN KNOWS EXACTLY HOW TO HELP HER CLIENTS BUILD, ACHIEVE AND MAINTAIN FABULOUSLY HEALTHY LIVES, WHATEVER THEIR EXISTING HEALTH CONDITIONS. SHE DOES THIS THROUGH PROVEN AND PERSONAL TECHNIQUES TO ALLOW HER CLIENTS TO ACHIEVE THEIR DREAMS.

BHBFITNESS.CO.UK

Chapter 9

MENOPAUSAL ROLLERCOASTER

By Helen Helliwell

We go from regularly or irregularly ovulating, safe in the knowledge that our bodies have the protection of those precious hormones, oestrogen and progesterone, to a roller coaster time of unpredictability in so many ways.

I was super blessed by seamlessly transitioning from a fertile, regularly ovulating woman of 54 years of age to a complete stoppage of those monthly joys.

No more storing sanitary protection, ensuring I had enough when going out, lots of toilet visits to check I was alright, especially in high-stress situations, and no concerns about unwanted pregnancies.

Indeed, my doctor informed me when I was 52 that I should be on hormone replacement therapy as I was the right age for menopause, and was amazed when I said I was still ovulating every month. However, this is so important, although I was very thankful for no night sweats, mood swings, weight gain, or other unpleasant symptoms, I did not think about the implications of post-menopause.

A lot of literature is written about menopause, the symptoms and treatments available.

The worries ladies have regarding the link between hormone replacement therapy and breast cancer is understandable, and it is not surprising if, like me, ladies sail through this period, they think all is well and are resistant to hormonal therapy afterwards, as I was.

I believed my health and fitness levels pre and during menopause were good enough to enable me to get through this period successfully and never gave much thought to afterwards.

So what changed? I did, aged 60.

Having been to the doctors to find out how my different hormone levels were changing, I was prescribed generic hormone replacement patches but found the difficulties of obtaining three months' supply and could not start without them.

Back to plan B – did I have one?

I then started researching the importance of ensuring any hormone replacement therapy was appropriate for individual ladies. I tried again with a private clinic, again being prescribed generic oestrogen cream, which proved very hard to measure accurately, progesterone tablets and female testosterone cream.

Was it easy to administer – definitely not – and I started to feel menopausal symptoms, including memory issues, lethargy, and mood swings. I was horrified this was happening to me at 60 years old.

It would have been easy to give up at this point – I had tried the regular routes – it had not worked, until I started this therapy – or so I thought.

However, the menopausal roller coaster, as it is for so many women, should not be this challenging if we understand more about our bodies.

So, I took a deep breath, restarted my research and found myself at another private clinic offering bio-identical hormone replacement therapy. I was at this clinic on another matter and found myself in tears over my situation, much to my embarrassment, as I am not usually overly emotional.

Thankfully, the qualified nurse talked to me about the many other ladies who had sat in the same chair, of all skills, from chief executives to homemakers, business owners to retired ladies, who had all felt a loss of control of their emotional selves and wanting balance back in their lives.

For the first time, I recognised my body was talking to me and submitted myself to blood tests, which was a big deal as I hate needles.

The tests were completed in America, with the results returned within a week. I was shocked that despite my previous attempts at hormone replacement therapy, my vital oestrogen, progesterone and testosterone levels were very low, indicating I was well into menopause.

Why did this worry me so much? Simply put, low levels of these hormones can trigger several serious health conditions, including potentially heart attacks and strokes.

Other conditions could also be triggered, and this scared me. It was the wake-up call I needed to recognise that my body needed the help of these vital hormones we take for granted when ovulating all those years.

We may not think of the downsides of losing the protection once we are in the menopause years.

It would have been very easy to celebrate not struggling with the symptoms of menopause and enjoy not having to use sanitary protection every month, dreading the first signs of menstruation, the tiredness, sore breasts, possible skin dryness and the need for intense personal hygiene. However, I realised how much it wasn't a cause for celebration. It was the opposite; the urgent need to recognise my body had served me well for the 54 previous years, and now it wanted my urgent help. Did I listen? Yes, I did.

My prescription was made up for my bio-identical hormonal therapy in an easy-to-use pump action bottle, pre-measured and rubbed into my skin twice daily. I will have my blood tests again in three months to ensure an accurate prescription and use a lifelong maintenance dose. Knowing prescriptions are plant-based means virtually no risk of breast cancer, and keeping up breast screening, bowel screening and cervical smears all ensure I am looking after my body.

It's so very important to me that this menopausal rollercoaster I have been through proved to me the vital need to look after my body after menopause, even when I had not suffered any issues pre-menopause or during menopause.

I believe it is so important we listen to our bodies throughout our lives, recognise that just because we do not have symptoms, it does not mean all is well, and have the courage to get correct tests done, accept the results and use the best possible treatments available to assist us alongside healthy lifestyles, appropriate food and drink and good exercise to keep our bodies strong, fit, flexible and happy.

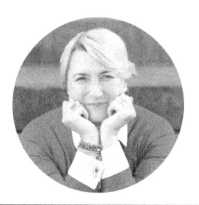

JO HOWARTH

JO HOWARTH IS AN ADVANCED HYPNOTHERAPIST AND MINDFULNESS PRACTITIONER. SHE RUNS THE HAPPINESS CLUB AND TEACHES PEOPLE HOW TO LOOK AFTER THEIR MENTAL HEALTH AND EMOTIONAL WELLBEING. SHE HAS TWO BEAUTIFUL DAUGHTERS, TWO GORGEOUS CATS AND ONE VERY NAUGHTY DOG.

THE HAPPINESS CLUB IS A MONTHLY MEMBERSHIP CLUB WHERE MEMBERS RECEIVE DAILY SUPPORT FROM, AND 24/7 ACCESS TO, QUALIFIED THERAPISTS. JO IS AN INSPIRATIONAL SPEAKER AND BESTSELLING AUTHOR OF 6 BOOKS. IN 2017 SHE WON TWO NATIONAL AWARDS FOR HER WORK IN THE HAPPINESS CLUB AND IN 2020 SHE WAS THE RUNNER UP FOR NORTH WEST ENTREPRENEUR OF THE YEAR, THE ONLY FEMALE FINALIST.

THEHAPPINESSCLUB.CO.UK
JO@THEHAPPINESSCLUB.CO.UK

Chapter 10

MY MENOPAUSE EXPERIENCE

By Jo Howarth

Ah, the menopause. There are so many things that nobody tells you, so many things you learn and experience.

As a teenager, I remember being vaguely aware of my mother going through "the change," as she called it. But as a teenager, I didn't want to know any detail about exactly what my mother's body was going through; I was far more preoccupied with whatever I was experiencing then. So I had virtually no awareness of the menopause other than it was a pain in the ass to experience.

I believe I was "peri-menopausal" for a good few years before I knew what was happening. I decided in my mid-forties to come off the contraceptive pill, and, quite frankly, all hell broke loose.

My lovely regular monthly periods were all over the place; I needed to track when they were supposed to appear or even if they might appear. They became heavier than ever and lasted twice as long as usual, and sometimes, they didn't come at all.

I felt tired. All the time.

I was exhausted and couldn't make it through a day without a decent nap around lunchtime. I thanked every god that had ever been created that I worked for myself and could manage my diary around these naps.

And then, one day, my entire body started aching, every muscle, from head to foot. The only place I felt comfortable was in a warm bath; I made jokes about becoming a mermaid because I spent so much time lying in water so that I didn't ache.

As a practising therapist, I already had a good daily meditation routine and mindset tools, for which I was eternally grateful. They helped me no end to navigate the changes in mood that I was experiencing and the brain fog that began to descend.

I went to my doctor, like any sensible person would, and was told it was probably all hormonal, but there was no point doing any blood tests because I hadn't been off the pill long enough, and anyway, hormone levels fluctuated so wildly throughout the month that one week it might show I was menopausal and the following week it might say I wasn't.

So, I decided I would have to investigate for myself. Around this time, a friend of mine, who had been through early menopause, posted a link to a list of the signs and symptoms of peri-menopause on social media.

What was this thing called peri-menopause? I just thought the whole thing was called the "menopause". I later discovered that menopause is just one day when you have not had a period for 12 months.

Anything before that day is peri-menopause, and anything after it is post-menopause.

But, back to the link my friend posted. It was an eye-opener. It listed all the symptoms below:

Hot flashes	Burning tongue
Irregular periods	Digestive problems
Fatigue	Muscle tension
Memory lapses	Allergies
Night sweats	Brittle nails
Loss of libido	Body odour changes
Vaginal dryness	Itchy skin
Mood swings	Osteoporosis
Panic disorder	Tingling extremities
Urinary tract infection	Insomnia
Bloating	Difficulty concentrating

Hair loss or thinning	Irregular heartbeat
Sleep disorders	Anxiety
Dizziness	Depression
Weight gain	Joint pain
Incontinence	Electric shock sensation
Headaches	

Oh my word, I cannot tell you how many pieces of the puzzle fell into place when I read that list!

That weird burning tongue feeling that had been concerning me.

The itchy head and arms that had me baffled.

I could eat the foods I had always eaten but was piling on the pounds like there was no tomorrow.

The dizzy spells that I had experienced for no apparent reason.

I couldn't remember the proper words for things or where I had left things. Asking my daughters to put the cheese back in the sausage (when I meant the fridge) and finding the loaf of bread in the plate cupboard caused laughter and concern.

When I read that list, there were only four things I hadn't experienced in the past year.

So, if my doctor wouldn't diagnose me, I would diagnose myself, I was peri-menopausal.

Realising that and allowing myself to acknowledge it helped me immensely. I doubled down on my meditation and self-hypnosis practice. I allowed myself those naps without the slight tinge of guilt accompanying them. I was generally easier on myself, and I started taking better care of myself.

But there were still a lot of symptoms to deal with, and I couldn't spend the rest of my life living in the bath!

I knew I didn't want to go down the HRT route. Rightly or wrongly, I just felt that it wasn't for me. I wanted to use a natural approach. I want to say that I researched the best and most holistic solutions, but the honest answer is that one of the women in my group of hypnotherapy trainees was a herbal medicine practitioner. We started chatting about my symptoms, had a consultation, and I started taking herbal medicine two or three times a day.

Within a relatively short time, my body aches were gone, followed swiftly by the fatigue, and even the weight gain stalled; although it would be a while before I started returning to my previous size and shape, I'm still working on that one.

Over time, most of my symptoms either stopped or lessened.

Sometimes, a new one would appear; I didn't have hot flashes; for instance, they developed a good couple of years in.

But every time something new happened, I would contact Hannah, my herbal practitioner, and she would prescribe me a new medicine to help. It didn't entirely get rid of every symptom, but I cannot begin to tell you how much it helped.

And then the big day arrived! I hit the menopause itself.

It almost crept up on me in the end, that fateful and momentous day. I blithely assumed that once that day was over, all the symptoms would be gone. I soon realised exactly how naïve that assumption was. My hot flashes and night sweats only started once I was post-menopausal.

So now I have moved into a place of acceptance with it all.

Sometimes, my symptoms flare up, and sometimes they die down. Sometimes, I have hot flashes, sometimes I'm a bit more tired than usual, and sometimes I feel as fit as a fiddle.

It can be painful and a pain in the ass. It can be difficult, and sometimes you wish it would just fuck off and leave you alone. But "the change" has also shown me how strong and capable I am; it has helped me learn to take each day as it comes, ask for help when I need it, and take good care of myself physically and mentally. And I will be eternally grateful for all of those things.

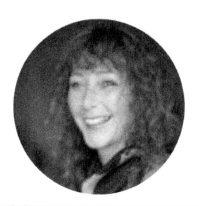

JUTTA WOHLRAB

JUTTA WOHLRAB IS AN ENTHUSIASTIC MIDWIFE COACH, TRAINER ,SPEAKER AND AUTHOR. SHE ENJOYS WORKING WITH WOMEN THROUGH ALL STAGES OF LIFE. HER WORKSHOPS HAVE INSPIRED WOMEN FROM ALL OVER THE WORLD TO TAKE THEIR LIFE BACK INTO THEIR HANDS.

AS A YOGATEACHER AND COACH SHE WAS THE FIRST ONE TO TEACH HORMONYOGA THERAPY IN AUSTRALIA .SHE HAS SHARED HER KNOWLEDGE AROUND WOMENS HEALTH FROM BODY AND MIND IN INTERNATIONAL CONFERENCES AND BEYOND. KNOWLEDGE IS POWER. KNOW HOW IS EMPOWERMENT .

JUTTAWOHLRAB.COM .
JUTTA@JUTTAWOHLRAB.COM

Chapter 11

THE POSITIVE POWER OF YOUR MENOPAUSE

By Jutta Wohlrab

You may wonder why I chose this title when I tell you that my menopause was quite a journey, but I want to share the amazing things I discovered along the way.

But first things first. I'm a midwife, coach, trainer, yogini, and all-round optimistic person. I was a feminist from an early age, became a professional midwife when I was twenty, and enjoyed a healthy lifestyle.

Looking back from the moment I celebrated my 60th birthday a few weeks ago, I was always interested in women's health and eager to find ways to feel good in body and mind. By the time I was well-established in my career, I thought I knew it all…

How wrong I was! In my mid-forties, I moved to Australia and started working in a birth centre. As well as my shifts at the centre, I taught pregnancy yoga, ran classes for expectant mothers, etc. My life was full, busy and happy, and I loved sharing my knowledge of birth hypnosis, nutrition, and Chinese medicine.

But then my periods stopped dead, taking me totally by surprise. On top of that, I had terrible migraines sleeplessness, and was careering around on an emotional rollercoaster. What was happening to me?

Somehow, it never occurred to me that this was the start of my menopause, and I searched for my lost periods. I did everything I could think of, including seeing a chiropractor and following a course of action that Chinese medicine recommended – which brought back a few very light periods – but that was it.

I was in shock, felt wretched, and was just all over the place. I couldn't understand what was happening, and the sleepless nights weren't helping – I couldn't even think straight.

One day, it finally dawned on me – could it be menopause? I had some blood tests done, and they confirmed my (rather belated) suspicions. I felt as if my life was over, and the GP, apart from some vague words of comfort, had nothing to offer in the way of practical advice. I was going to have to help myself.

Balance your body

First, I had to make changes to get myself back into balance again. These were the first steps I took, and they have worked for me and many others:

- Change your diet: If you are a meat-eater, vegetarian for a few months.

- Cut sugar from your diet completely.

- Eat lots of fresh fruits and vegetables, especially things like grapefruit, chicory, asparagus, radishes, sprouts, cabbage – anything slightly bitter, as it will help stimulate your liver energy.

- Broccoli, apples, peaches, and carrots can positively impact your oestrogen levels; soybeans, tofu, chickpeas, legumes, fish and meat mimic oestrogen in the body.

- Reduce your coffee intake as coffee is dehydrating.

- Steer clear of red wine: it will drive your energy up but also bring hot flushes, night sweats and headaches.

- To kickstart these changes, it might be helpful to put alcohol, spicy food, sugar and coffee on hold. (Don't worry: this phase will not last forever.)

- Take linseed oil daily to keep inflammation down.

Embrace your second spring

I'm afraid I have to disagree with the lie that the media peddles to us: that we're old, unattractive, and ideally invisible. I would be whoever I wanted to be and do whatever I wanted to do.

The menopause can give you much freedom (not least to have sex without the fear of becoming pregnant). You can turn into a tigress and decide to ride the dragon of your menopause – that's what I chose to do.

I knew the time had come to make some major changes. Working shifts was doing me no favours, so I quit my job, went back home to Germany to care for my elderly parents – and started my own business.

This is your opportunity to free yourself of the pressure of doing what society expects you to do. The menopause offers you the chance to live up to your full potential. Take it from one who knows:

'So many women I've talked to see menopause as an ending. But I've discovered this is your moment to reinvent yourself after years of focusing on everyone else's needs. It's your opportunity to get clear about what matters to you and then to pursue that with all of your energy, time and talent.'

- Oprah Winfrey -

Taking it further

There are many more techniques, treatments and therapies to help you make the most of your menopause.

• Taking natural hormone supplements and the herbal treatments recommended by Chinese medicine.

• Having a course of acupuncture.

• Doing a simple breathing exercise like the following will bring calmness into your system: breathe in for a count of 4, hold your breath for 6, and exhale for 8.

• Getting some coaching to help build a positive mindset, eliminate stress, and focus on new opportunities.

Yoga

By a stroke of luck, when I returned to Germany, I found that Dinah Rodrigues, the creator of hormone yoga therapy, was running courses there. I did the training and was amazed to see its effect. With regular practice of only 10 to 15 minutes a day, women could increase their estradiol levels by 150% over a few months. Soon, I began offering these courses in Germany and Australia.

Women loved these courses and the results they achieved – one woman told me that after only two days of training, she had gone to a party and received lots of attention and compliments…

* * *

The menopause is a crazy yet empowering time, so find a like-minded community and start enjoying your second spring!

www.juttawohlrab.com .

jutta@juttawohlrab.com

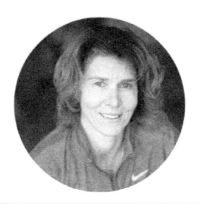

LISA CHADWICK

LISA IS A SELF-EMPLOYED PERSONAL HEALTH AND FITNESS TRAINER, WORKING WITH WOMEN OVER 40, BOTH ON A 1:1 BASIS AND ONLINE.

SINCE QUALIFYING OVER 20 YEARS AGO, SHE HAS SPENT THE BEST PART OF HER CAREER HELPING LADIES FEEL FITTER, STRONGER AND MORE CONFIDENT BY CHANGING THEIR LIFESTYLES. SHE NOW SPECIALISES IN WORKING WITH MENOPAUSAL WOMEN, AS SHE CAN RELATE TO THE MANY ISSUES FACED DURING MIDLIFE AND HOW EXERCISE HELPS TO ALLEVIATE THESE PROBLEMS.

SHE PRACTICES WHAT SHE PREACHES WITH A SIMPLE APPROACH! SHE WORKS WITH THEM, NOT FOR THEM AND CONSTANTLY ENCOURAGES AND MOTIVATES.

MOTIVATES.ME.UK
LISA@MOTIVATES.ME.UK
LISA@MENOMIDLIFE.ORG.UK

—

Chapter 12

GET ACTIVE, FEEL GOOD, EMBRACE MIDLIFE

By Lisa Chadwick

You may wonder if exercise can help you deal with menopause, and if so, how?

Let's look at some benefits of regular exercise during menopause, which will help counteract many symptoms you may experience during midlife.

Menopause is an important transitional period in a woman's life that prompts physical, mental and emotional changes. Because menopause is life-changing in all these ways, it is an ideal time to start looking after your body and mind through health and fitness. Creating a regular exercise routine is a fabulous way to feel more energised!

Here are a few potential benefits:

After menopause, you may be at risk of heart disease due to lower oestrogen levels.

Regular cardio exercise can help to reduce this risk.

Menopause can sometimes contribute to insomnia. Exercise may encourage better sleep patterns.

The hormonal changes during menopause can affect your mental health.

Exercising regularly can release "happy hormones" called endorphins, which help relieve menopause symptoms, making irritability and mood swings easier to cope with.

A substantial loss of oestrogen can affect the health of your bones, but resistance exercises can help support your bone and muscle health and keep them strong.

So, how much exercise should you do before and during menopause, and what exercises are best?

Adults should do some physical activity every day, but even before embarking on any new fitness routine (especially during menopausal changes or if you have medical conditions or any concerns), it is always best to speak to your GP first. Make sure your activity and its intensity are appropriate for your fitness.

According to the *NHS 'Live-Well' Guidelines (2023)*, adults should aim to:

Do strengthening activities that work all major muscle groups (legs, hips, back, abdomen, chest, shoulders, arms) at least twice a week.

Do a minimum of 150 minutes of moderate-intensity activity or 75 minutes of vigorous-intensity activity a week, and spread exercise evenly over 4 to 5 days a week or every day.

Reduce time spent sitting or lying down and break up long periods of not moving by introducing some activity.

Consider incorporating additional movement during your day, like squatting or standing on one leg as you brush your teeth!

If you're not sure where to start with exercises that are ideal for women going through menopause, then here are some ideas:

Hormone Balance and Bone Health

Due to the loss of oestrogen, which has a massive impact on our bone health, strength training is vital to help balance the decline in hormone levels.

Menopause significantly speeds up bone loss and increases the risk of osteoporosis. Research indicates that up to 20% of bone loss can happen during midlife, and approximately 1 in 10 women over the age of 60 are affected by osteoporosis worldwide (*Endocrine Society, 2023*), so strength training can help increase muscle mass and strengthen the muscles around naturally declining bones to protect them.

One of the effects of oestrogen decline is an increased risk of sarcopenia (the loss of muscle mass specifically related to ageing). This may lead to osteoporosis, which can cause other issues with your bones, such as the risk of fractures. To start with strength exercises, you could do bodyweight exercises such as squats, planks, or push-ups (from your knees if it helps), lifting kettlebells and dumbbells, or even using fixed resistance-based gym machines.

Weight Maintenance

Weight gain is a common symptom of menopause.

Swimming or water aerobics are easy on the joints, using the entire body and are another fantastic way to burn calories. Cardio exercise can also increase your energy levels, boost your mood, and enhance your sleep quality. Some examples of cardiovascular exercise include dancing, cycling, high-intensity interval training style workouts and running/jogging. Any activity will help maintain a healthy metabolism, too.

Balance and Mobility

Maintaining your balance as you get older is important to reduce your risk of falls. Balance and mobility can decline during menopause, again due to loss of muscle mass. Another advantage of these types of exercises is that they usually involve a mind-body aspect. This means that they can reduce stress levels. Yoga or Pilates are ideal practices for balance, mobility and anxiety.

Elevate Your Mood

Try walking, which is the simplest form of low-impact exercise. Of course, whilst walking promotes good cardiovascular health, consistently walking 20-30 minutes daily, for example, can boost energy and mood. Being amidst nature is a great boost for your general well-being.

Anxiety and Depression

For many women, menopausal symptoms make us realise that our body is changing, which can be stressful, not to mention all the other challenges midlife can throw our way. Yoga can be such a powerful practice for the mind during menopause, and if you have joint or muscle discomfort, you may prefer this form of low-impact exercise.

Working out with friends is a great way to boost mood and socialise, which is helpful when ladies often experience more anxiety and a lack of confidence. Find a friend with similar fitness goals and work together towards achieving them.

There have been a lot of studies to support exercise as a tool to reduce anxiety and depression in older adults, although there is still more research to be done in this area.

So, you can see why it is so important to **get active** during menopause. However, before you embark on any fitness regime, do what feels best for *you* and *your* body - do something that makes you **feel good!** If you choose a form of fitness that you enjoy, you will more easily boost your mood and are more likely to stay motivated and consistent.

Perhaps commit to a fun challenge that will help motivate you, and remember to appreciate and love your body as it is right now, **not** where it was in your 20's!

Any exercise, whether a strict routine of lifting dumbbells or a gentle stretching routine, is beneficial. Never discount taking short, brisk walks, doing housework, or gardening, which we class as *NEAT *(*Non-Exercise Activity Thermogenesis.)* It is all good practice!

If you are not currently active, finding time to exercise can seem like a challenge, but you must try to do something and fit it into a daily routine.

Set yourself up for success by having *realistic* goals and go from there. Always seek advice from a Personal Trainer if you need help with movement patterns or exercises.

Remember... Movement is key! Movement is good! Embrace midlife with energy!

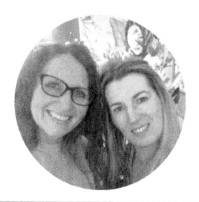

RACHEL YOUNG
CAT ROBINSON ARMOR

QUICKLY DISCOVERING A SHARED DETERMINATION
BETWEEN THEM, THAT MENOPAUSAL YEARS ARE A
TIME FOR A TRANSFORMATIONAL UPGRADE AND
NOT A TIME TO BE MISERABLE.
BRINGING TOGETHER YEARS OF EXPERIENCE,
TRAINING AND EXPERTISE IN MENOPAUSE,
NUTRITION, ALTERNATIVE MEDICINE,
PSYCHOTHERAPY, HYPNOTHERAPY AND MORE,
RACHEL & CAT CREATED THE MENOPAUSE WEIGHT
LOSS UPGRADE SYSTEM.
THIS ENABLES WOMEN TO DITCH THE MISERY OF
MENOPAUSE, LOSE WEIGHT, AND EMBRACE THE
BENEFITS OF IMPROVED SYMPTOMS, PHYSICAL AND
PSYCHOLOGICAL HEALTH, SELF-WORTH, AND
CONFIDENCE.

RACHEL@MENOPAUSEMIND.LIFE
INFO@THEHORMONEFAIRY.CO.UK
FB GROUP:
THE5DAYMENOPAUSEHEALTHYHABITSCHALLENGE

Chapter 13

BACK FAT AND JELLY WOBBLES

By Rachel Young & Cat Robinson Armor

Everywhere we look, adverts and articles claim the ultimate solution for quick weight loss or a miraculous transformation.

These quick fixes are appealing, and these diets sell largely because people desire miracle results without the hard work.

This is not surprising as we are told that dieting is a struggle, that we must deprive ourselves and will be miserable and hungry until we reach a magic number on the scales, and only then will we be happy and fulfilled.

When we are already juggling so many challenges, including a whole array of menopausal symptoms, it makes sense that we desire a quick resolution to weight gain, wanting to move swiftly to the place where we are promised ultimate slender confidence and joy.

Alongside dubious psychology used for selling weight loss dreams, what many of these diets fail to address is the whole picture.

During perimenopause to post-menopause, so many changes are happening in our brains that we can feel powerless and out of control.

So, to address weight loss and other symptoms we must consciously take back that power and control by making choices and changes for ourselves.

We need changes that re-establish external and internal balance for long-term sustainability and longevity and changes that align with what our mind and body require for health and nourishment. For this, a holistic approach is needed.

This re-establishing control and balance process involves ditching old unhelpful habits, beliefs, thoughts, and behaviours contributing to weight gain and symptoms. In their place, embracing habits, beliefs, thoughts, and behaviours that nurture us.

We can do this by starting exactly where we are now and making a series of simple step-by-step changes at the right pace.

Neema's Story (aged 48 in perimenopause)

Neema came to see us for weight loss support, dejectedly stating, "I'm all back fat and jelly wobbles." She explained that she had tried many diets, and none were working; she was gaining weight at "an alarming rate", which was affecting her mood and marriage.

We asked Neema questions about; her home and work life, intimate relationships, friendships, support systems, symptoms of perimenopause, moods, diet, exercise, self-care, hydration, sleep, habits, behaviours, historical trauma, grief and loss, goals, aspirations, and beliefs about herself, others, and the world.

She kept a food and drink diary, paying particular attention to what was driving her to eat and drink (was it hunger or something else). Additionally, she recorded her thoughts, feelings, moods, events, and observations, whether food-related or not, in a daily journal.

What we discovered

- Neema's sugar intake was high, and her water intake was low. She substituted breakfast and lunch with milky coffee. Feeling "peckish" at around 3 pm, she began snacking. At 6 pm, she would eat a healthy meal with her family.

- When her family were all in bed, she experienced cravings that were "never satisfied".

- She felt "too exhausted to exercise".

• She was experiencing high-stress levels, hot flushes, aching joints, mood swings, was self-critical, tired all day, and woke feeling "depressed and exhausted".

• She described her relationship with her husband as "strained" and her social life as "non-existent".

• Her confidence was "lost", and she felt lonely.

• She wanted to lose enough weight to fit into her favourite dress and find purpose in her life again.

How we worked with Neema

We created a step-by-step plan for Neema using The Menopause Upgrade Weight Loss System. This system uses five keys that we have found to be essential for successful change and sustainable weight loss, health, and nourishment during menopausal transition.

Key 1 Education

Understanding why weight gain in menopause is happening is essential for feeling more empowered and in control. We encouraged Neema to share her learning with her husband, family, and friends so she could begin to build a support network.

Some areas we shared information on were why women gain weight in peri menopause, the role of hormones, the impact of stress, poor sleep, nutrition, hydration and exercise, the importance of a support system and of acknowledging her needs with compassion.

Key 2 Psychological health

Our deeper mind is exceptionally powerful; it was important that Neema's subconscious mind was working in alignment with her conscious wants, needs and desires of weight loss, confidence, purpose, and health.

We taught Neema to reconnect with her hunger signals and focused on her self-worth, purpose and confidence, with breath work for stress management.

Journaling identified negative thought patterns and beliefs around food, with conscious challenging of unhelpful beliefs, feelings, thoughts, and behaviours.

Hypnotherapy supported the creation of new healthy habits, improved sleep and addressed emotional eating. Inner child healing work relieved the emotional burden of loss and grief reducing her psychological stress load.

Key 3 Physical health

As Neema's stress load was high, and she was struggling with body aches, it was important to introduce exercise at a manageable level.

Neema began by setting herself a daily steps target, which she increased over time.

Key 4 Culture and beliefs

We can carry guilt, judgement, and shame around our experience of being a woman. These, often deeply buried and isolating feelings can create an extra stress load on our mind, hindering weight loss and the emergence of our sense of value, worth and confidence.

Neema disclosed guilt for wanting to change her life and a belief that "others" expected her to "always put everyone else first as a dutiful mother and wife".

Neema shared these revelations with her husband and was relieved to understand that he did not share her belief-driven assumptions. Interestingly, she described this discovery as "a great weight off my shoulders".

Key 5 Resources

Having access to the correct information, support, dietary advice, planning and tracking records tailored to the uniqueness of every woman's menopausal experience is essential for weight loss success, the reduction of symptoms and the rediscovery of confidence and purpose.

Creating simplicity, clarity, and accountability for Neema through relevant resources was vital to reducing stress and overwhelm; it was also psychologically rewarding as she could experience and celebrate her progress at every step.

The Outcome

Over six months, Neema achieved her goal of dropping two dress sizes.

She felt healthier and energised, with improved sleep and clearer skin. Her mood was balanced, and her aches were mostly gone.

The most rewarding part for us was seeing the sparkle in her eyes when she spoke of her future aspirations. Neema had discovered her new purpose.

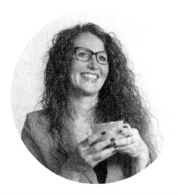

RACHEL YOUNG

RACHEL IS THE FOUNDER OF MENOPAUSE MIND AND PHOENIX HYPNOTHERAPY AND COUNSELLING SERVICES. SHE IS AN EXPERIENCED PSYCHOTHERAPIST, HYPNOTHERAPIST, SPEAKER, TRAINER, AND COACH. WITH OVER 30 YEARS OF WORKING IN MENTAL HEALTH AND EDUCATION, SHE IS NOW BASED IN BEDFORDSHIRE, WHERE SHE LIVES WITH HER FIVE CHILDREN AND WORKS WITH LOCAL, NATIONAL, AND INTERNATIONAL CLIENTS.

WITH THE BELIEF THAT MENOPAUSE IS A TIME OF UPGRADE AND TRANSFORMATION, RACHEL IS DETERMINED TO CHANGE THE MENOPAUSE CONVERSATION. SHE HAS BEEN FEATURED ON BBC NEWS AND THREE COUNTIES RADIO AND HAS SPOKEN FOR NUMEROUS ORGANISATIONS, INCLUDING HEALTHCARE PARTNERSHIPS, LOCAL AUTHORITIES, COCA-COLA, AND LOCAL BUSINESSES.

WWW.MENOPAUSEMIND.LIFE
RACHEL@MENOPAUSEMIND.LIFE

Chapter 14

MENTAL HEALTH, TRAUMA AND MENOPAUSE

By Rachel Young

Mental health struggles are a common and often overlooked experience of the perimenopause to post-menopause transition.

We know that hormones have a role to play here, but what is often not considered is the impact that childhood trauma, emotionally charged past experiences, and unresolved grief can have on the severity and duration of symptoms.

Who is at risk?

Individuals with a history of anxiety, depression and challenging mental health are potentially more at risk of experiencing mental health symptoms during menopausal transition.

It is also the case that individuals who have never struggled with issues around mental health and emotional wellbeing can be floored with debilitating anxiety, fears they are going mad, new phobias, depression, sadness, rage, paranoia, negative thinking, loss of confidence, and the list goes on.

Suppose you have experienced trauma, grief, emotionally challenging life experiences or have lived with negative self-beliefs and not had the opportunity to heal from these experiences. In that case, the menopausal transition is when old unresolved feelings and thoughts can become known again.

This revivification of old traumas and the emergence of unhelpful beliefs can negatively impact your emotional wellbeing from mild to completely debilitating.

I don't know who I am anymore

As a psychotherapist, I have had the privilege of working with numerous wonderful women. Women who have been rocking life with successful careers, a happy family life, good friendships, an active social life, and strong intimate relationships. That is, until they hit perimenopause, it's as if all they have known, worked for, and focused on no longer makes any sense.

Women describe themselves as feeling stuck, lost, lonely, confused, and powerless. Questioning their purpose and relevance in their relationships, families, careers, life, and the world. They are no longer trusting their own bodies and minds and are losing their sense of worth, value and confidence. "I don't know who I am anymore" is a common phrase I hear.

A time for change

Whether women have a history of mental health symptoms or are experiencing them for the first time, the menopausal transition is unquestionably a prime time for change.

Changes in our brain, hormonal and physical changes are undeniably happening. So, the key is finding new ways to listen to and respond to these changes, discovering ways to take control and feel in control rather than the out-of-control experience so many women have.

*During the transition from perimenopause to post-menopause, it becomes **essential** for good mental and physical health to find new ways of thinking, behaving and being.*

Unburdening your mind and body

Part of this process of change and taking control is creating the space to work through old traumas, giving due attention to past and current loss and grief, releasing stuck anger, and engaging in the compassionate healing of psychological wounds.

This healing process lifts a huge stress load from our brain and body and releases debilitating emotional burdens that we have been heaving around, sometimes for decades.

We don't necessarily have to forgive or accept that what happened to us in our lives was okay, but for our mental health and wellbeing, we need to be able to release the power that old psychological wounds have held over us.

When we do this, we put ourselves into a place of choice and control, creating space and the right environment for our new and emerging selves to flourish.

Once we process emotional trauma and rid ourselves of old, non-serving beliefs, our future aspirations will often look very different from those of pre-menopause.

This can be challenging initially (*especially for those of you who have gone through life as people pleasers or over-givers due to a sense of not feeling good enough in some way*) as it can become necessary to have a clearing out phase.

The clearing-out phase

When creating positive psychological change for ourselves, embracing new and healthier beliefs, and stepping into our true selves as women, it can become evident that some parts of our lives and environment no longer fit with who we are.

Ending relationships that emotionally drain us and creating distance from people who don't support our worth and value may be necessary steps to take. Putting self-protecting boundaries in place, saying no to others, and saying yes to yourself can take practice. However, in doing this, you will soon discover the life-changing benefits to your mental health, physical health, and life fulfilment as you make new rewarding friendships and experience the emotional freedom of living a life that aligns with your true self.

Your time to upgrade

Experiencing mental health symptoms in the menopausal transition can be highly challenging. You can feel completely alone; no one understands, and nothing is helping.

What I am about to say next might feel like a stretch if you feel this way, so bear with me while I explain.

Please consider the time from perimenopause to post-menopause not as a design fault or a time to be endured or feared but as a time to be embraced and celebrated. It is a time to upgrade yourself to live your best and healthiest life.

It is a time when our deeper mind communicates very loudly that something is wrong.

Symptoms demand that we take a hard look at our past and current burdens, our inner selves, our lifestyle, our environment, our mental and physical health, our relationships, and our time past, versus our time left.

When we begin to take action to unburden our mind and body from historical and current psychological stress loads that no longer serve us, we become emotionally unshackled, releasing space and energy for creativity, our natural intuition, freedom of choice and a robust sense of self-worth.

A robust sense of self-worth is a cornerstone of good and balanced mental health and can enable us to celebrate our time from perimenopause to post-menopause as an opportunity to grow into what we truly want, need and desire.

When fostering psychological balance and health, we naturally feel, think, and behave in ways that support our wellbeing. Helpful hormones are produced, and a more harmonious environment, within which the natural hormonal changes of menopause can take place, is established. This results in fewer and milder symptoms increased mental and physical energy, and a non-negotiable determination to embrace the wonderful power of womanhood.

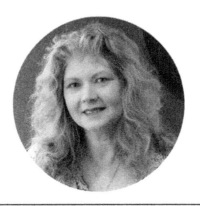

RITA PRESTON

RITA PRESTON BEGAN HER WRITING CAREER IN EARNEST DURING THE GLOBAL PANDEMIC IN 2020 AND LEFT THE INCOME TAX PROFESSION AT THE END OF 2021 (AFTER 32 YEARS) TO PURSUE WRITING FULL-TIME.

WITH THE PUBLICATION OF MENOPAUSE: WHAT NOBODY TALKS ABOUT! RITA IS THRILLED TO COUNT THIS CHAPTER AS HER 9TH COLLABORATIVE BOOK PROJECT!

RITA'S RECENTLY RECEIVED ACCOLADES ARE THE 2021 GOLDEN QUILL AWARD WINNER FOR A.B.A.T.E. OF PENNSYLVANIA AND AS AN AMBASSADOR FOR MO2VATE MAGAZINE, RITA'S WRITING IS BLOSSOMING JUST AS SHE DREAMT OF AS A CHILD IN PRIMARY SCHOOL.

HER FIRST SOLO BOOK, MY LIFE IS A MEME, WILL BE RELEASED IN EARLY 2024,

RITA@RITAPRESTONSVIEWS.COM

Chapter 15

SHE'S HOTTER THAN HELL!

By Rita Preston

Menopause. The dreaded progression of female life. Hot flashes. Mood swings. End of child-bearing. That's the tip of the iceberg.

Even after eons of women experiencing 'the change,' we still dread talking about it. There are hundreds of jokes, especially for husbands dealing with their wives.

Ultimately, menopause is no joke.

I remain baffled about the actual term. In my experience with linguistics, it is a 'pause' of menses. It is not a pause. It is the end of menstrual cycles and the ability to produce offspring.

Menopause itself is brief. It occurs when a woman experiences her very last menstrual period. She won't even know with certainty until 12 months have passed (per my now-retired gynaecologist).

Even if periods cease for 11 months but return on month 12, menopause does not occur. For a woman experiencing mood swings, that adds one more state of confusion!

As young females, many look forward to our first period – we will achieve womanhood! We become women!

Then, reality hits. We are still teenagers (give or take, depending on our hormone levels and physique), and our parents have no problem reminding us that we are still 'children' and live under their roofs as their dependents.

More reality arrives. Every month. Sanitary products. Cramps. Mood swings. Bloating. Food cravings.

What was once longed for, waited for, and something we celebrated becomes monthly drudgery. Periods can last for a day, a week, or anything between, and sometimes even longer. Some of us can predict our cycles like clockwork.

Others know it's a constant guessing game and carry our sanitary products with us daily because we never know when we'll get a bloody surprise in our undergarments.

How awful, that a week of cramping and bleeding, signals we can give birth to fellow humans, is known as a curse! Being able to procreate is amazing! Sometimes, we get to skip cramps and bodily tenderness – hooray!

There comes a point when we look forward to menopause so that we no longer have to deal with the work of 'that time of the month': keeping clean, sometimes hourly maintenance, and dealing with food cravings, discomfort, and mood swings.

Wait a minute!

That sounds like menopause: food cravings, discomfort, mood swings, hot flashes!

My family started the hot flash symptom of menopause early, decades before menopause.

My family doctor said I was too young when I started 'flashing' in my 30's. I reminded him about my female relatives who were his patients and to review our charts collectively.

We start early and drag out everything! We started greying our hair in our 20s on my mom's side of the family. Why would menopause be any different?

My poor husband.

We will celebrate 34 years of marriage this summer, and he's still putting up with my slow, unmethodical progression into post-menopausal womanhood. For decades, we've had a running joke that I treat him like a Greek god, giving him burnt offerings when I cook meals! (I concur! He's my personal gourmet, and I cook merely to survive.)

He has always said that I'm "hot stuff". Little did we know how 'hot' I would become as I age! (He has also joked that my thermostat has always been broken...)

Hot flashes sneak up when least expected. At this point in my life, they seem part of my daily routine.

I dress in layers, carrying a winter coat in the car in case I cool off, and I wish there were more layers to shed in the summer months!

One physician recommended I cut back on coffee and alcoholic beverages. That would help reduce hot flashes. WHO, in their right mind, tells a middle-aged woman to give up caffeine and alcohol? I guarantee my sour mood will elevate!

I officially 'changed' several years ago. I'm only 59 and refuse to be considered old.

Life does not end with menopause. I have much yet to do! I have grandchildren with whom to play, motorcycles to ride, travel adventures to make, and a husband to love!

Physical changes create emotional changes. Some are good; some are downright ugly for those around us.

I regret when I've been grumpy, when I've allowed negative emotions to spill forth, and when I've stressed out those I love.

The women in my family get a look on our faces (when we're tired, angry, not thinking….) – dubbed the Go-To-Hell look. I'm told I have a top-notch version!

Can I change the times I've been rude, mean, and ugly? No. All I can do is strive to improve myself, seek medical help when needed, and work on being a better me. This is a work in progress: not glaring at people, working on my innate quick hot temper, and apologising with sincerity.

My husband has been an angel in putting up with me as my female body and cycles changed (even though I sometimes thought he was a jerk).

He's still with me. Note: My husband is not a jerk! He's wise and diplomatic (most of the time). He is human, too and kind.

Men change over their lifetimes **too**, and our world doesn't discuss that much. Not enough medical attention is provided for men going through puberty and experiencing their mid-life changes.

The world has come a long way in recognising the transitions of women. We need to do the same for men.

We joke that I was my husband's mid-life crisis (he was single when I met him, but we have a 17+ year age difference).

He said he got a hot wife instead of a hot car! I am blessed he has stuck with me as I work my way through the many changes of life.

I am thankful that he tolerates me when I put a car window down in the middle of winter to cool off while he's cold and needs the heater – and I'm ready to pass out from the heat, triggering another flash!

It's cool that he still says I'm 'hot stuff'!

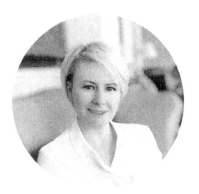

SHARON BROWN

SHARON IS FOUNDER AND PUBLISHING
CONSULTANT AT THE AWARD WINNING
PUBLISHING COMPANY, THE BOOK CHIEF (THE
PUBLISHERS FOR THIS BOOK).

SHARON RUNS VARIOUS BUSINESSES INCLUDING
MO2VATE MEDIA (AN ONLINE BUSINESS AND
INFORMATION HUB) AND THE SPEAKERS INDEX (A
PUBLIC SPEAKING DIRECTORY AND MAGAZINE).
SHE IS ALSO A BUSINESS MENTOR FOR
SANTANDER'S WOMEN'S BREAKTHROUGH
PROGRAMME AND HAS RECENTLY BEEN
APPOINTED BOARD DIRECTOR FOR A
NATIONWIDE WOMEN'S CHARITY.

SHARON IS A WOMAN CURRENTLY GOING
THROUGH MENOPAUSE!

THEBOOKCHIEF.COM
MO2VATEMEDIA.COM
SHARON@THEBOOKCHIEF.COM

Chapter 16

A FASCINATING PHASE

By Sharon Brown

I've found the menopause journey challenging but also fascinating. You're acutely aware of everything going on, and it almost feels like it's some endurance test, a bit like the Krypton Factor (if anyone remembers that!)... You pass through each obstacle only to hit the next one.

Then that passes, and you're onto something else. I've not had one symptom that has lasted seven years. Each year seems to bring a new test, challenge or experience.

Until you experience it, it all seems unreal and unbelievable, as if it's not happening and it's all in your head.

Thankfully, I think I'm coming to the end of my journey (at least I do hope so), but the past seven years have gone in the blink of an eye, and during the first few years, I didn't even realise I was in peri-menopause. I started noticing changes in my body and mood around 46.

I'd always been very active and fit with an athletic build with my weight never more than around 10'4.

I had also been blessed with 'young looking' genes (thanks, Mum and Dad!), so although I had been warned that weight gain would be harder as menopause approached, I didn't take much notice.

I'd been able to lose weight very quickly in the past when I needed to. My confidence to keep doing that would soon prove futile.

Achy joints started annoying me early on. I felt itchy, too, which I couldn't understand. I noticed cellulite had begun to appear, and my skin and hair had changed. My hair especially was so frustrating… it had always been fine hair, but when styled, it looked good. Now, I looked like a scarecrow. It was dry, and I couldn't do anything with it. Even after a haircut, it stuck out in all the wrong places. I spoke to my hairdresser about it, and she confirmed that many women had complained about the same thing, so I didn't feel so freaky!

The achy joints were starting to keep me awake at night, and then, in 2019, I had the start of a frozen shoulder. This is another strange condition as you don't realise what it is until you can't move. My mum had both shoulders frozen during her 50's, so I know the journey I was in for. It was not until recently that I realised this can be caused by menopause, too.

With a frozen shoulder, you are paralysed and can't do much, and you'll try everything and anything to get rid of it.

unfortunately, there is no quick fix. It makes you desperate... I visited a physiotherapist, a chiropractor, and the Doctor. I had steroid injections, cupping, Acupuncture... you name it, I did it, but nothing helped. Deep Freeze proved to be the only thing that gave me relief. It can last up to 3 years, and I wouldn't wish it on anyone. It's the most pain I've ever felt, and I hope never to be repeated.

Thankfully, mine was solved in six months due to a fall where my arm went in the opposite direction, thanks to having a naughty kitten at the time.

I passed out with the pain, but within two weeks, I realised my shoulder was starting to come out of a 'freeze'. I was one of the lucky ones in that situation as my mum suffered terribly with hers and eventually had to get a 'manipulation' under anaesthetic, which is excruciatingly painful.

After this, lockdown came, so my active lifestyle seemed to come to a standstill. The weight piled on, and I'm two stone heavier three years later than I was. Lifting it now feels impossible, so I'm riding the storm until I'm out the other end. Then, I'll take serious action to get some of the old 'me' back.

One of the things that I rarely hear being talked about is the feeling of absolute despair that you can feel. This hit me like a fast-moving train, and being someone who doesn't suffer from depression, I didn't know how to handle it.

If you're reading and feeling this, I'm not trying to scare you. Just to help you understand, this is also a symptom of changing hormones and one that will pass.

My menopause journey has taken on many different phases, each lasting its course and then moving on to something else.

The despair stage lasted around six months. Each month, for about 24 hours, my happiness evaporated, and a dark cloud of hell overtook me. It's within this period that you need to be aware and also be careful of your thoughts. Try and remember that this too will pass, that it's a temporary drop in something within your body that makes you feel what I can only describe as suicidal. I felt utterly lost, worthless and devoid of all other emotions except that my life meant nothing and would be better off not in existence.

Shake that feeling off... talk to someone. Many women do commit suicide during menopause, and I suspect a lot to do with these very feelings.

It did pass.

The latest stage of my journey has been the most challenging, which is also surprising considering the other things. I've started to experience extreme hot flushes and sweats. They were very sporadic beforehand and not often, but then, all of a sudden, I was heating up with a furnace inside me every half hour.

My pores open, and water comes out. It's not like normal sweating… It's as if you've walked into a hot sauna for about 60 seconds, and then the feeling starts to dissipate.

Currently when writing this, I've had this for three months, and then just two weeks ago, it stopped suddenly. What that means, I have yet to learn. I don't know if it's coming back or if it's telling me that my period is ending soon. Incidentally, I hadn't had one for 63 days and thought it was gone; then it appeared out of the blue again and was very heavy. Still no more hot flushes at the moment, which is great.

I found the latter very challenging as it hits you anywhere. You could be in a meeting, on a call or anywhere. It doesn't care! It makes you feel flustered. You lose your train of thought, throwing you off kilter whatever you're doing. You're hot, sweaty and want to change your clothes constantly. I don't know how people live in countries that have 40 degree heat every day… I would die!

Brain fog has been prevalent probably more during the 'middle' period, where a wall comes down, and you go completely blank! I think this has passed now.

These things can feel scary when you're unsure what to expect, but like everything in life, nothing lasts forever. It's a journey that we all need to go through and an awakening period in our lives.

Even though I've had challenging times with these symptoms and life in general, I've also thrived through it in other ways. The key is to talk to others. Learn and understand as much as you can to know the steps to improve these symptoms.

It's not a death sentence. Embrace your newfound self and know you'll be like a new woman when you reach the other end! I'm starting to feel 'like me' again and can't wait to start this new stage in my life.

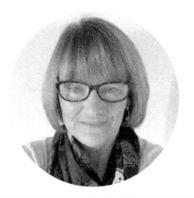

SUE COPELAND

SUE'S BACKGROUND IS IN GENERAL NURSING, WITH OVER 35 YEARS OF NHS EMPLOYMENT AND A WEALTH OF PUBLIC HEALTH EXPERIENCE, SKILLS AND KNOWLEDGE.

SHE SUPPORTS MENOPAUSAL WOMEN, HAVING UNDERTAKEN ADDITIONAL TRAINING IN THIS AREA. SUE HAS ESTABLISHED AND FACILITATED AN EXTREMELY SUCCESSFUL AND INTERACTIVE INTERNATIONAL MENOPAUSE FACEBOOK GROUP (CURRENTLY OVER 6000 MEMBERS). SHE BELIEVES IN HAVING A POSITIVE MINDSET AND REGULARLY PRACTICES MINDFULNESS AND MEDITATION ALONGSIDE OTHER EFFECTIVE STRATEGIES. SUE LOVES SEEING THE POWER OF THESE IN ACTION AND SUPPORTS OTHERS TO WORK ON CREATING A MORE POSITIVE MINDSET TOO. SUE IS A STRONG BELIEVER THAT CHANGE HAPPENS AT THE END OF OUR COMFORT ZONE.

MENOMIDLIFE.ORG.UK
SUE@MENOMIDLIFE.ORG.UK

Chapter 17

HELP! MY WAIST HAS DISAPPEARED

By Sue Copeland

As our key hormones (particularly Oestrogen) start to decline in the run-up to menopause (peri-menopause), our bodies compensate for this by storing it in fat cells, especially the ones around our middle, which explains why we often notice our tummy getting bigger. Excess weight around the tummy can lead to sugar, carbohydrate cravings and an increased appetite.

Our bodies compensate by producing a type of Oestrogen called Oestrone from our adrenal glands and fat cells. This leads to the laying down of fat, especially around our middle. However, this does protect against osteoporosis, brain, and heart disease – so it is not all bad!

Other potential reasons for putting weight on at this stage of life include:

● A history of fad diets, which rarely lead to long-term weight loss.

● Moving less due to achy joints, burning up less energy.

- Our body needs less energy as we age, but we often continue to eat the same.

- We lose muscle mass too (sarcopenia), and less muscle = less calories burnt = weight gain. Yo-Yo dieting leads to more muscle loss too.

- We may have less to occupy our minds as families grow and leave home.

- We may be caring for elderly relatives, putting additional stress on us.

Nutrition during Menopause

Nutrition/Hydration Tips:

It is crucial to balance your blood sugar as much as possible – low blood sugar triggers the production of stress hormones. Avoid eating sugary snacks, processed foods, and carbohydrates, e.g., white bread/ rice, which can lead to spikes in blood sugar.

Eat complex carbohydrates, which are rich in fibre, provide sustained energy and assist with the digestion and metabolism of foods.

Protein is essential during midlife; it helps with reduced muscle mass and bone density.

It supports blood sugar balance by slowing down the release of sugars into the bloodstream, reducing sugar cravings and helping us feel fuller for longer, too.

Limit your intake of alcohol and caffeine, which can have a diuretic effect. Staying hydrated - drinking water, especially before meals, can lead to you eating fewer calories. Aim for 6-8 glasses daily.

Serve yourself smaller portions, and avoid skipping meals and grazing between meals.

Ensure your food is full of nutrition to protect your health and help weight control, choosing more fresh fruit, veg, oily fish, nuts, seeds, whole grains, and white meat. Keep a food diary.

Intermittent Fasting / Time Restricted Eating

Some find this approach helpful in achieving weight loss. In this case, you eat within a set period, e.g., 12 hours and fast for the remainder of the day, e.g., 12 hours. This is called the 12:12.

The theory is that our bodies move into a repair stage, which can support health and weight loss.

Exercise

Excessive abdominal work will not immediately help you lose weight around your tummy area but will strengthen your abdominal muscles. A layer of fat will hide these unless a mix of aerobic workouts, strength training and a sensible, healthy diet are incorporated into your fitness regime.

Each person's body has a natural pattern of where fat is distributed - some people lose fat from their stomachs first, while others get slimmer hips. This is often genetically programmed.

Your body will decide where to store the fat, and your lifestyle determines how much it stores.

So, can you turn fat into muscle? The simple answer is no.

Turning fat into muscle is physiologically impossible, as muscle and fat comprise different cells.

Exercise Tips:

• Move every day; it does not have to be excessive.

• Make a fitness plan, including low/medium intensity cardio, including walking at a pace you feel is working your heart and lungs.

Swimming, cycling, strength/resistance training; working with weights or resistance bands to help maintain muscle mass and bone density (around 2-3 times a week if you can), mobility, flexibility, balance, and core work.

Sleep - Can sleep affect weight loss?

Yes, it can! Poor sleep (often common during menopause) makes the body inclined to store calories as fat. It triggers the body to produce more insulin and cortisol. Higher levels of these hormones prompt our bodies to store energy as fat, especially in the abdomen.

Poor sleep slows down our metabolism and makes it work less effectively, leaving more unexpended energy to be stored as fat.

Poor sleep also increases appetite, leading to hormone changes that regulate hunger and the feeling of fullness. It can also lead to cravings for high-fat/calorie foods.

Research by Sleepstation (2023) found a link between poor sleep and weight gain.

Stress

The relationship between stress and weight

Feeling stressed can lead to food cravings – where you are likely to eat out of seeking comfort rather than feeling hungry. Commonly eaten foods are chocolate, biscuits, ice cream, cakes, salty snacks, higher fat, and sugary foods with little nutritional value.

When under stress, your body releases cortisol, which interferes with metabolism.

The stress hormone cortisol encourages abdominal fat deposits. If stressed, you may find you are eating the same amount of food but not burning off as many calories as you usually do.

Here are some lifestyle tips for reducing stress:

• Schedule exercise into your weekly routine.

• Practice self-care – reading, hobbies, a relaxing bath, and listening to music.

• Do not over-commit, promising to be everything to everybody.

- Start a Yoga/Pilates class.

- Practice Meditation/Mindfulness.

- Take a social media/IT break.

- Talk through your problems with someone willing to listen.

- Seek professional help when necessary.

- Take time to get outdoors in nature.

- Address those areas that are causing you anxiety and stress.

Mindset

Mindset is as important as choosing the right foods, exercising, reducing stress and improving sleep when it comes to weight management.

Six tips for improving your mindset:

1. Use affirmations, which help reprogramme your beliefs such as 'I choose healthy foods to support my weight loss journey.'

'I am grateful to have a body capable of exercising".

2. Visualise your ideal weight – how do you look and feel? What has changed in your life?

3. Focus on the positives – the delicious healthy foods you will eat; get creative in the kitchen. What will be gained by being your ideal weight?

4. Make small, consistent changes rather than great, big ones that you are unlikely to stick to.

5. Keep a journal – record your success, note compliments you receive, and note any changes to your body. Look back at your journal when you feel less positive/motivated.

6. Try hypnosis downloads for weight loss, these can support behaviour/belief changes as well as being relaxing.

In Summary:

Many factors affect your weight, especially during menopause. Anything is possible with dedication, support, a strategy, goals, willpower, and accepting that slip-ups may happen!

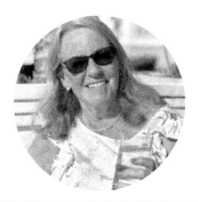

SUSAN BEESLEY

SUSAN IS A DEDICATED ADVOCATE FOR WOMEN'S WELL-BEING AND IS PASSIONATE ABOUT EMPOWERING WOMEN AGED 50 AND BEYOND.

THROUGH HER LEARNED PERSONAL EXPERIENCE, SHE SHARES HER WEALTH OF KNOWLEDGE AND EXPERTISE, SPECIALISING IN GUIDING WOMEN THROUGH THE TRANSFORMATIVE JOURNEY OF MIDLIFE. SUSAN OFFERS HOLISTIC SOLUTIONS TO CONQUER MENOPAUSE SYMPTOMS NATURALLY AND INSPIRES WOMEN TO EMBRACE THIS UNIQUE PHASE OF LIFE WITH VITALITY AND CONFIDENCE.

SUSAN ENCOURAGES WOMEN TO PRIORITISE SELF-CARE, NOURISH THEIR BODIES, UNLOCK THEIR INNER RADIANCE AND EMBARK ON A TRANSFORMATIVE JOURNEY TO SURVIVE AND THRIVE IN LATER LIFE, LOOKING AND FEELING GOOD ABOUT THEMSELVES.

BEYOND50MENOPAUSE.COM

Chapter 18

THE "JOYS" OF MENOPAUSE AFTER 50

By Susan Beesley

The "Joys" well, maybe not!

Menopause is a natural part of ageing that usually occurs as a woman's oestrogen levels decline with symptoms lasting up to four years after a woman's last period, but to quote, "*varies depending on the individual*."

With more than seventy reported symptoms of menopause, it's hardly surprising our individual stories are as diverse as our symptoms as a recent interview between Lisa Snowdon and Nihal Arthanayake on Radio 5 Live highlighted.

I am writing this to you at 68 years of age, having fully expected the symptoms to have all but disappeared, so I can only guess I'm one of the unusual individuals...

Or am I? From the stories I'm hearing, it would seem not!

This is my menopause story, and I hope that by reading it, you will find your light at the end of the tunnel and know that if you are still experiencing symptoms, there are ways to deal with them naturally.

So, let's backtrack for a moment…

I had my children in my late twenties and knew that two was all I wanted, so I had no worries as I approached my forties that my childbearing years would end. Having re-married and acquired three step-children, I was happy to see this new phase of life approaching…

So, it was a bit of a shock when it arrived because suddenly I was heaped with some unexpected issues that no one had thought to tell us about if we're honest…

Certainly not if you were born in the 1950's as I was!

But it's OK, as I was told, the common symptoms like memory lapses (*known as brain fog today*) and poor concentration are very common, as are hot flushes, night sweats, low mood, difficulty sleeping…

But don't worry; they will only last 4 or 5 years!

I was 50 and remember the day clearly.

I was in France up in the mountains on a skiing holiday with friends and woke up to what would be my last period, although I didn't know that at the time.

Nothing very unusual, and I hadn't had any of the usual peri-menopause symptoms I had heard about from friends (*I didn't even know there was a name for it back then*)

I considered myself very lucky if this was the end of all *that* *"woman stuff."*…

What I wasn't to know was what was coming next.

The sleepless nights, hot flushes, moods worse than the pre-menstrual ones and more to come.

Yikes!

I remember discussing it with my Mum one day, and she said it's best to just put up with it because she had HRT (*Hormone Replacement Therapy*), and it changed her life… and not for the better, given the weight she gained and hated.

Hardly surprisingly, there was no way I would look at HRT as a solution if that was a side effect.

So, I put up with it for years and years and years.

My poor husband, the things he had to put up with.

We often need to remember how this affects our partners and family.

I remember reading an article recently where the actress Viola Davis was talking about what she describes as "The Hell of Menopause," describing it as a "*dark hole*" and one where she, on any day, will either love her husband or want to kill him.

How I can sympathise as I've been there too!

And let's not talk about sex!

Now, not everyone will have the same symptoms, and some will not have any at all. I've talked to a lot of women since I began sharing my story on TikTok (Beyond50Menopause) and Facebook (LivingYourBestMidlife)

And by far and above all, other symptoms are weight gain (*most of us call it our "meno belly"*), mood swings and poor sleep.

That was me, too – I began to put on weight around the middle even though I was active, enjoyed my yoga, going to the gym and eating sensibly.

Why?

So, I did what most people do, I tried weird and wonderful diets… but they don't work, do they?

Over the years, the weight crept up until a health check revealed I had put on 20 lbs. I was forced to do something about it after being diagnosed with familial high cholesterol and given a stern warning about the potential for a stroke or heart attack.

Definitely enough to get my attention!

I discussed with my consultant my next steps, and she suggested I start following a Mediterranean-style diet, taking regular exercise (*walking daily*), and taking regular medication for the high cholesterol, which I reluctantly agreed was necessary.

However, I didn't want to take anything for my menopause symptoms despite her recommendation to take HRT, and that led me on a journey and a mission to find natural alternatives to HRT.

There's a plethora of information to sift through, but one thing I concluded was that going on unrealistic restrictive diets to lose weight and enrolling at the gym to try and get rid of the belly and that unwanted fat around the middle was not the answer…

Because you have to get to the source of the problem.

And I did.

It's not your fault you're having trouble losing weight at this time of life, because it's entirely due to our hormonal changes, we're laying down fat and exercise and diet alone will not solve the problem.

I wanted to put this into perspective and help other women have a better experience of menopause as naturally as possible, give them some background and clarity and share the things I've discovered along the way…

To offer some natural solutions to those things that affect the weight we put on during menopause. The truth is that when our hormones are out of balance, our life is out of balance.

Your MOOD (stress hormones)

Your DESIRE (sex hormones)

Your WEIGHT (metabolic hormones)

I discovered that they all influence each other, and our many different symptoms are interlinked.

I put to the test a plan that involved natural supplementation to balance mood and sleep and added that to the things I know will help you lose weight naturally - exercise and diet.

Why?

Because moving your muscles and lungs will mobilise the fat stores and switch on the feel-good endorphins, and eating the right nutrients at the right time will switch on your gut microbiome and activate your mood and metabolism.

Then you add SLEEP.

Your secret fat-destroying weapon.

Getting good quality sleep on top of a good healthy diet and daily exercise and you will start to see the pounds and inches melt away (literally).

Now, it's not going to happen overnight, but I'm happy to say that it worked for me, and I've seen it working for others going through the same challenges in their life.

I'm happier and healthier, and life post-menopause is looking up!

In another chapter, I'll talk more about the benefits of holistic management of menopause symptoms and how Ancient Chinese Herbs are today responsible for improving our health and wellbeing.

Chapter 19

A HOLISTIC APPROACH TO POST MENOPAUSE WEIGHT GAIN

By Susan Beesley

The truth is I was desperate to find a natural solution, and I did find myself down a lot of rabbit holes in the early days of research, but I was determined to find a holistic approach to dealing with my worst menopause symptom – the dreaded "menobelly."

The more I read and researched, the more determined I was to get to the bottom of it, but it was reading an article by Dr. Shawn Talbott* about what's known as the gut-brain-axis that confirmed I was on the right track. *Dr Shawn Talbott is a Psychonutritionist, renowned author of The Cortisol Connection and Mental Fitness which highlight why we put on weight around the middle and story belly fat.

To put this in perspective, did you know that your gut is responsible for far more than you may have imagined and that many of the health issues we have today relate to your gut biome (the millions of bacteria that live in your gut and regulate your body)?

I didn't either.

Could this discovery help me with the unexpected weight gain, and was there a holistic solution?

It seems it could, so I dug a little deeper…

Here I was at 68 post-menopause, as are many other women I talk to, and the factors that lead to our weight gain during menopause are still in effect after menopause, and, sadly, it won't miraculously disappear when menopause ends!

Also, because of our body's changes during menopause, the lifestyle approaches that once limited weight gain (*exercise and diet especially*) may no longer have the same impact.

With that said, having a healthy diet with a variety of plants, sleeping well, and exercising can help make managing your weight easier after menopause, but what goes on in your gut can influence your weight gain, so we want to keep your gut healthy.

I want to share a little of what I discovered so that you can decide whether holistic supplementation is for you.

I am not a doctor or have any scientific or medical background, so none of what I am sharing should be considered medical advice.

It's just my research to help you understand your body better and how you can turn things around if you are open-minded to something different.

Let's talk a bit more about the gut then, how it is intricately linked to the period of life we know as the MENOPAUSE and why it is possible to manage our symptoms holistically.

When you reach menopause (around 50), your ovaries have stopped producing sex hormones (*progesterone and estrogen*).

Now, this is where it gets interesting because it's these sex hormones that affect our gut bacteria. Given that these hormone levels are changing our gut microbiome, the effect is some very familiar symptoms - hot flashes, night sweats, mood changes and weight gain.

For post-menopause women, weight gain is one of our major health concerns, and if we're honest, we know it has far-reaching consequences, so not only do we want to deal with it from a health perspective, but we want to look and feel good too, don't we?

The good news is that we can now modify the gut microbiome and find holistic solutions.

Enter the world of ancient Chinese herbs and plants.

Women have commonly used medicinal plants and herbs to manage menopausal symptoms and improve their overall quality of life for a very long time; we just haven't been exposed to their benefits in the Western world.

Could that be the answer I was looking for?

I trawled through many articles and looked at different herbs and plants that can be used to manage the symptoms of menopause. I've read many of them to understand their role, and ultimately, they have helped me choose the supplements I take today.

Going back to the gut and knowing we need to manage our gut biome during and post-menopause, the first herb was Ashwagandha.

Ashwagandha, also called Indian ginseng, has been used in Ayurvedic medicine for centuries and is ideal for supporting our stress response system, helping lower and restore cortisol levels, regulating estrogen and progesterone levels and lowering inflammation in the gut.

It enhances mood and focus, improves stress management, supports healthy energy levels and promotes mental wellness.

When our hormone levels are balanced, then we can tackle the elephant in the room - weight gain - because, as you can see, everything is interlinked.

If you can manage your gut biome naturally as I do now, you will sleep better, your mood and anxiety will be managed, and those imbalances that lead to storing fat will be dealt with, too.

I discuss this in more detail in my chapter "The Joys Of Menopause After 50."

You can now manage your menopause naturally from the inside out.

That's just one example; books have been written on ancient Chinese medicines, herbs and plants, and if you are like me and want to do what you can naturally, you should research.

What to look for in a holistic supplement?

Make sure it is 100% natural and not a synthetic version – start with a probiotic supplement that can introduce specific strains of beneficial bacteria into your gut – those that contain strains that have been studied for their effects on gut health, such as Lactobacillus and Bifidobacterium species.

Don't rely on supplements alone – incorporate natural ingredients and foods into your diet that help support a healthy gut microbiome during this phase of life.

Fiber-Rich Foods such as whole grains, vegetables, fruits, legumes, nuts, and seeds are in your diet.

Fermented Foods rich in probiotics such as yogurt, kefir, sauerkraut, kimchi, miso, and kombucha.

Prebiotic-Rich Foods that provide nourishment for beneficial gut bacteria. Foods like garlic, onions, leeks, asparagus, bananas, and oats.

Omega-3 Fatty Acids are found in fatty fish (like salmon, mackerel, and sardines), flaxseeds, chia seeds, and walnuts, all of which have anti-inflammatory properties that can support gut health.

Polyphenol-Rich Foods - plant compounds with antioxidant and anti-inflammatory properties. Foods like berries, green tea, dark chocolate, and red wine

Turmeric and Curcumin are known for their anti-inflammatory effects

Ginger: Ginger has anti-inflammatory and digestive benefits. It can help soothe the digestive tract and promote a balanced gut environment.

Of course, the list goes on and on, but now you know that you can manage your menopause naturally and finally tackle your weight gain holistically.

We now know many effective natural options to help women not just "endure" menopause (*hot flashes, night sweats, mood fluctuations, weight gain, loss of libido, etc.*) but to thrive through menopause and into their later years.

Don't let anyone tell you otherwise!

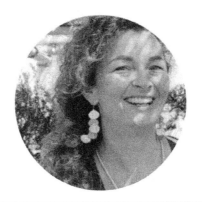

SUZANNE LAURIE

SUZANNE IS A MIDLIFE/MENOPAUSE COACH AND EMOTIONAL AND BINGE EATING SPECIALIST.

HER SPECIAL INTEREST IS HELPING MIDLIFE WOMEN NAVIGATE A HEALTHY AND HOLISTIC MENOPAUSE, FIND FOOD FREEDOM AND BUILD A CONFIDENCE IN THEIR BODIES THEY HAVE NEVER EXPERIENCED BEFORE.

SUZANNE HOLDS A BSC (HONS) IN NUTRITIONAL THERAPY AND AN MSC IN POSITIVE PSYCHOLOGY AND IS A CERTIFIED COACH. SHE HAS OVER 20 YEARS OF EXPERIENCE AS A PRACTITIONER AND TRAINER OF NUTRITION AND COACHING PROFESSIONALS AT ONE OF EUROPE'S LEADING PRACTITIONER TRAINING INSTITUTES.

MOTHERFLUSHINGMIDLIFE.COM
SUZANNE@MOTHERFLUSHINGMIDLIFE.COM

Chapter 20

THE ROLE OF 'INFLAMMAGING' IN MENOPAUSE

By Suzanne Laurie

It must be important when a word gets the 'RomCom' and 'Brunch' treatment. Although this fusion of the words 'inflammation' and 'ageing' may not sound as glamorous as 'KimYe,' it holds significant importance for menopausal women, as it may worsen ALL their symptoms.

Inflammation is an essential immune process. When you sustain an injury, it supports healing; when you're fighting illness, it helps combat invading pathogens. It even supports the body's day-to-day business, helping clean up waste products and debris created by the metabolic reactions that keep us alive.

However, there's a catch. Inflammation should be short-term and easily switched on and off like a light. If it persists, even at low levels, or is excessive in specific body areas, problems arise.

Chronic inflammation leads to the breakdown of healthy tissues and cells and triggers the production of free radicals (highly reactive molecules that can wreak havoc in the body).

Your immune system then needs to continuously clean up this mess, perpetuating more inflammation...and a vicious cycle begins.

Inflammation, Ageing and Gender

In younger years, our bodies have a remarkable ability to balance damage and repair.

However, cumulative damage can overwhelm the immune system as we age. Interestingly, this tipping point is commonly observed around the age of 50, a time when many women are in the thick of menopause.

This correlation is no coincidence, as oestrogen is a powerful natural anti-inflammatory. So, when levels decline leading up to menopause, we are reliant on the body's other anti-inflammatory mechanisms, topped up by dietary anti-inflammatories.

Consequently, women in the menopausal transition and beyond become vulnerable to low-level chronic inflammation, which helps explain common symptoms like joint pain and increased allergies and the increased risk of chronic health issues such as heart disease, arthritis and dementia after menopause.

According to the inflammaging theory, modern Western lifestyles play a significant role in premature ageing and chronic disease. Inflammation has a particular affinity for collagen, a vital protein in connective tissues that provides structural support to our skin, cartilage, joints, bones, and tendons. When inflammation attacks collagen, it can reduce the quality and duration of our lives. Sorry, but there's no sugarcoating that.

And if we've enjoyed some of life's more hedonistic pleasures over the years (even if it's a dim and distant memory), things may catch up with us sooner and with more force!

Even those sleepless nights with babies, toddlers, and snoring husbands take their toll. And let's not forget the constant juggling act you're probably still doing between work and family life, possibly washed down with a nightly glass of wine.

However, understanding the connection between inflammation and ageing empowers us to take proactive steps towards mitigating its effects.

By adopting a healthy lifestyle, managing stress, and making informed choices, we can find that inflammation/anti-inflammatory balance is required to reduce menopause symptoms and increase health and longevity.

Addressing Inflammation

Oestrogen will decline during menopause, but it is not our only anti-inflammatory; the body is designed to adapt and survive.

Having it at very reduced levels does mean the immune system's army is a woman down, though, so providing additional anti-inflammatory resources becomes vital.

Luckily – Mother Nature offers everything we need in foods packed with potent anti-inflammatory compounds. Recent research indicates that regular healthy lifestyle choices can slow the progression of, and even reverse, common inflammatory conditions (Dimitrov et al., 2017).

However, it's important to be realistic. Sometimes, the fun things in life do come with a side of inflammation. Also, your job and family commitments may not allow for a constant state of zen! But you need to know that to offset the damage this causes; you must ensure a daily dose of anti-inflammatory foods and lifestyle choices.

Top anti-inflammatory foods:

The following foods contain abundant anti-inflammatory and antioxidant phytonutrients, which dampen down inflammation in the body and help protect it from free radical damage.

- **Fatty fish** rich in omega-3 fatty acids, such as salmon, sardines, and mackerel
- **Berries** such as blueberries, strawberries and raspberries
- **Leafy greens** such as spinach, kale, and collard greens
- **Herbs and spices**, particularly turmeric, black pepper, basil, garlic, ginger, cardamom, cayenne, chamomile, coriander, cinnamon, cloves and rosemary
- **Extra virgin olive oil**
- **Nuts** such as almonds, walnuts and hazelnuts
- **Tomatoes** are high in the antioxidant lycopene, especially when cooked
- **Green tea**
- **Dark chocolate** (at least 70% cocoa)
- **Beetroot**

Eating a rainbow of whole foods (red, orange, yellow, purple, green, white/brown) is vital to keeping the immune system healthy. Try to include some (not all) of the following daily – fresh fruits and vegetables, nuts and seeds, fermented foods (such as live natural; yoghurt, kefir, kimchi and sauerkraut), oily fish, high-quality oils, herbs and spices (go heavy!) and even a bit of dark chocolate.

It's easier than you think - live yoghurt with fruit and nuts for breakfast and a large salad (olive oil and herb dressing) for lunch or dinner will get you far.

Top Anti-inflammatory Lifestyle Habits

Regular moderate-intensity physical activity:

Outdoor exercise offers more potential for relaxation, stress reduction and vitamin D dosing (hugely crucial for immune health). And it's never too late to start. Just three months of moderate exercise can lower inflammation in previously sedentary older adults (Woods et al., 2012)

Prioritising quality sleep:

As key systems and organ repair happen at night. Hormone-induced night sweats and insomnia hinder this – so you may need to focus elsewhere if sleep disturbances are an issue. However, reducing inflammation can help significantly!

Stress-reducing practices:

Such as meditation, deep breathing, yoga, or mindfulness practices. Stress promotes inflammation by releasing stress hormones and triggering immune responses that can result in chronic inflammation.

Maintaining a healthy weight:

Excess weight increases inflammation as fat tissue produces and releases pro-inflammatory molecules.

Limiting alcohol consumption:

Alcohol disrupts the balance of gut bacteria, impairing the immune system and triggering the release of inflammatory mediators.

Staying hydrated:

Dehydration compromises proper blood flow, reducing the body's ability to remove inflammatory by-products and deliver anti-inflammatory compounds to affected areas.

Avoiding environmental toxins:

Including cigarette smoke (from smoking or passive smoking) containing high levels of chemicals that create extensive free radical damage in the body.

***

So, If you want to keep a spring in your step and your skin, reducing inflammaging is a must for years to come. It is also relatively simple, with just a few dietary and lifestyle changes. Remember – chocolate is on the list of anti-inflammatory foods, after all. Trust me, your body will thank you, it's worth it (and so are you).

Chapter 21

MENOPAUSE: ONE OF MANY MIDLIFE TRANSITIONS

By Suzanne Laurie

Menopause significantly transforms every woman's life, bringing multiple potential physical and psychological symptoms.

Whilst I am by no means underestimating its impact (trust me - I'm in the thick of it), it is just one element of our midlife journey that shouldn't overshadow other significant shifts that often occur simultaneously.

Indeed, midlife is like a magnet for change, with a variety of physiological, psychological and social stressors clustering at this time (Thomas et al., 2018).

Change can be a positive force, nudging us towards new challenges, but it can also come with company. Amid transformation, we often find loss.

Loss in Midlife

Generally, when we think of loss, our mind goes to the death of a loved one, but in reality, it arrives in many other forms during midlife – failed relationships, career changes, health challenges (our own and older relatives), children leaving home, downsizing and even our sense of identity. All whilst riding a hormonal roller coaster and watching bits and pieces shrivel, droop and drop off.

Even the relief many women feel when their periods finally stop may be bittersweet, as we recognise our reproductive years are officially behind us and, therefore (according to our youth-obsessed culture), we're now past our prime. Therefore, if we're not careful, grief can become an unwelcome and often unrecognised companion in our daily lives, bringing uncomfortable emotions that become difficult to shake.

For example, at 45, I'd been running my own company for 17 years, leading a fantastic team with my husband and raising two children together. Fast forward one year, and our business failed, leaving us with a combined income of absolutely zero. Our marriage quickly followed, and my husband moved to another country, leaving me as a full-time single parent.

As I write this, just 6 months have passed, so I'm still licking my wounds. I have days where I feel lost, lonely, scared and angry.

But, and it's a big but….I already see the bright side; I know I will be ok; I already am…most days.

So, what has got me through watching my life crumble before my eyes?

Resilience.

What is resilience?

In a nutshell, it's bouncebackability! – our capacity to respond to, withstand, adapt to and recover from adversity and challenge. If you are looking for one of the keys to happiness and positive wellbeing in midlife, look no further (Suss et al., 202).

And boy, does midlife (and menopause) require us to flex that resilience muscle, as it's often women juggling multiple roles (worker, partner, carer, friend) whilst becoming increasingly invisible in societies that laud female youth and encourage us to spend precious time, money and energy fighting the natural ageing process. But when I look around me, I don't see a throng of midlife women resigned to sitting out a miserable second chapter of their lives or succumbing to the real pressures they are experiencing.

Instead, I see pillars of strength carrying significant war wounds yet seeking new adventures. Why- because these women have resilience.

Can you build resilience?

But were they born with it? Can that be me, you ask? Yes, it can. Whilst resilience is in some part 'genetic', research shows it is modifiable and ebbs and flows with life's challenges (Bonanno et al., 2015). But, like most things worth having, we must proactively nurture resilience, particularly when life throws its best shots at us.

So, how do you build resilience?

Trust me- it's not as complicated as you might think! For my MSc, I studied all the research I could find to help compile a list of key factors that support resilience in midlife women. Here's what I found:

• Good physical health, supported by positive health behaviours (a nutritious diet, physical activity and sleep in particular)

• Strong social support (friends, family and/or an intimate relationship. Although all three are not required!)

• A positive outlook and optimism about the future

- Self-belief and a sense of self-worth

- Meaning and purpose

- Adaptability

- Faith….in being part of something bigger than ourselves

- Employment/financial security

The good news? They are primarily modifiable, and not all need to be in place to increase resilience. However, the more proactively we focus on some of them, the more likely we are to weather those midlife storms. If some feel like a stretch right now, don't worry - I'm offsetting my current financial crisis and perimenopause symptoms with a bucket load of healthy eating, optimism, and social support.

Interestingly, whilst my research suggested that menopause can have a mildly negative impact on resilience, it was not found to be a significant factor for most women unless they had severe symptoms. And this book will have you covered for the 'how to' of how to keep those to a minimum!

What does resilience look like?

Despite the mention of optimism and positivity above, it is not powering through with a brave face (no toxic positivity here folks).

Resilience can be raw, snotty and uncomfortable because it involves acknowledging, accepting and allowing ourselves to feel those challenging emotions without guilt or shame.

It's leaning on friends for support. It's saying no to commitments when you need to be alone. It's knowing that 'this too shall pass' and that there is a positive future even if you can't feel or touch it in the present. My research showed that most importantly- it knows that you are worthy of that future and that your knockbacks do not define you. They add to the knowledge and resolve you need to reach it.

And the really good news?

If you learn to ride those midlife and menopausal waves, the blows that leave us winded and scarred also make us happier long-term. Yes – we need to feel the grief, anger, physical symptoms and tedium to recognise and appreciate life's joys. If we can bounce back from the lows, we feel the highs more fully and for longer.

So, if you feel you don't have the strength you need to cope, or you'd like to be stronger in the face of menopause or other midlife challenges – I know you can be. Heck, you probably already are.

Revisit the list above and pick one thing today you can work on. Because, like every midlife woman looking towards the future, you deserve it to be bright and opportunity-filled. You've earned it.

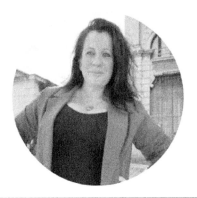

TABBY KERWIN

TABBY KERWIN IS A MULTI-AWARD WINNING MINDSET COACH AND ENTREPRENEUR, BEST-SELLING AUTHOR AND SPEAKER.

TABBY WAS ORIGINALLY TRAINED AS A PROFESSIONAL MUSICIAN AT THE ROYAL NORTHERN COLLEGE OF MUSIC AND LATER WENT ON TO STUDY FOR A MASTERS IN POSITIVE PSYCHOLOGY. SHE IS DEDICATED TO HELPING PEOPLE PERFORM AT THEIR BEST WHILST PRIORITISING WELLBEING AND PROTECTING THEIR MENTAL HEALTH AND REGULARLY TRAINS, FACILITATES AND SPEAKS ON THE SUBJECTS OF GRIEF, MENTAL HEALTH AND SUICIDE PREVENTION.
A FAN OF CHALLENGES AND HELPING OTHERS, IN 2023 TABBY CLIMBED MOUNT KILIMANJARO IN AID OF GRIEF AND MENTAL HEALTH CAUSES.

MODEFOR.CO.UK
THEPERFORMEXPERIENCE.COM
MODEFOR@GMAIL.COM

Chapter 22

FIGHTING THE MIDLIFE ODDS TO PERFORM AT YOUR BEST

By Tabby Kerwin

Whilst I am a positive psychologist, speaker, best-selling writer and award-winning mindset coach specialising in mental health and suicide prevention, I want to talk to you as me: Tabby Kerwin – woman, mum, widow, CEO and at the time of writing, living with peri-menopause.

If I told you there was a huge correlation between menopause and mental health issues, would you believe me? With all its physical effects that are more widely talked about, such as hot flushes and weight gain, you could be excused for not at first connecting the dots between poor mental health and even suicide and menopause... but we need to.

Connecting the dots between my mood and age got me curious that I could be experiencing peri-menopause... and my intuition was right...I had no other symptoms, but I knew this wasn't depression again, something I'd previously lived with.

According to the Office of National Statistics (ONS), in the UK, the rate of suicide in women aged 45-54 has increased by around 6% in the last 20 years.

Furthermore, in women, the age-specific category with the highest rate of suicide is 50-54 years old – slightly older than the most common category for suicide in men, which is 45-49 years old.

So, what's going on here… why is this age group that coincides with the most common age for peri-menopause and menopause experiencing this increase in mental health issues and suicide?

The most common suggestions are empty nest syndrome and menopause. That makes me statistics gold – widow, peri-menopause and empty nester! Yet, women are often treated for their low moods and poor mental health with medications for depression as opposed to HRT.

Now, I'm not here to suggest that anti-depressants shouldn't be prescribed; every woman's needs are different, but with such a connection between the ages of menopause starting and the increase in suicide, we have to look at the causes of low moods first, which could well be linked to menopause before we jump to a prescription of depression medications?

I was 44 years old when I first started noticing symptoms – but it wasn't the well-advertised hot flushes, night sweats, brain fog, stopping periods or lack of interest in sex that alerted me to my perimenopausal years – it was my change in mood.

I had previously lived with depression and anxiety for a decade as a younger woman, so I am no stranger to feeling those sensations of grey and numbness. I even experienced suicidal thoughts at that time, albeit fleeting, and they have never returned.

I am recovered now, and my recovery is dependent on me taking daily action to promote positivity, managing my emotions and being happy – and even in the wake of grief following the death of my husband Simon in November 2018, I stayed 'above the line' on the mental health continuum and emotionally fit – flourishing even.

It takes work, but it's part of my daily routine to do that work. My resilience and emotional fitness levels are high.

But a few years ago, I noticed a lethargy in my mood and low feelings when there was no real reason to feel that way, and I was doing the work on and for myself… so I got curious. Whilst I could feel my mood lowering, it wasn't the same grey and numbness I felt with depression – this was subtly different – but I knew I had to explore the emotions and feelings to manage them.

Honestly, I didn't know much about peri-menopause or menopause, but at 44, I was a way off that, wasn't I? Besides having a Mirena coil implanted, I wouldn't even know if my periods had stopped because I don't get them! I had no other symptoms of mid-life hormonal changes – just this mood issue got me curious!

I did my research (I'm a passionate learner – one of my tonic strengths!), and I concluded that the strongest possibility was that it wasn't a recurrence of depression, but in fact, it was the start of peri-menopause… and so, I started to treat it as such. Allowing myself some self-compassion and kindness for the natural changes and embracing Mother Nature's fun!

Over the next year, a few other symptoms emerged for me – some flushing and occasional night sweats and a change in bodily shape and weight despite doing all the good things regarding nutritious eating and exercise. That wonderful shift in how I hold my weight, which now revels in sitting across my stomach region – it's newfound place of comfort – I'm starting to embrace it, but it takes real work not to resent it!

Menopause does not exactly extend the hand of kindness, but you know what they say: *"Keep your friends close and your enemies closer."* Peri-menopause became my friend – it was doubtless here to stay, so I switched my mindset to embrace it. A change in mindset is a powerful tool for dealing with issues head-on and helps us to PERFORM at our best.

At this stage, I haven't needed to explore medical prescriptions yet (never say never), but boosting vitamins, especially vitamins B, C and D, Magnesium and Calcium, has had a positive impact on me at the same time as eating Oestrogen rich foods and switching up my exercise regime – much more strength and flex as opposed to pure cardio.

The biggest thing that has helped me PERFORM at my best has been focusing on my mindset. Embracing this chapter and working with it. Extending self-compassion to myself even though my body has changed and loving it in this new form – that's hard and a work in progress, but I'm getting there!

At this age, it feels like the odds are stacked against us like Mother Nature has a different agenda, and the statistics around mental health and suicide tell a huge and sad story of lives lost.

But maybe, if we embrace those changes in emotions and moods and treat them with the kindness they deserve and we get curious about the possibility that peri-menopause or menopause could be the cause, not just dismissing it as a diagnosable mental health illness, we could not only start to flourish in our lives, we could also begin to save other lives.

Your mindset is everything - so choose to embrace the fabulousness of midlife, roll with it and get curious.

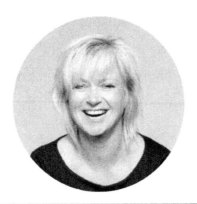

TRUDI ROSCOUET

TRUDI DECIDED TO REQUALIFY AS A MASTER PERSONAL TRAINER SPECIALISING IN WOMEN AND CHILDREN'S FITNESS AND OBESITY IN 2010.

THE WORD "MENOPAUSE" NEVER ENTERED HER VOCABULARY AT THAT POINT AS SHE THOUGHT HER 50-YEAR-OLD LADIES WHO COULDN'T LOSE WEIGHT WERE NOT DOING WHAT THEY WERE TOLD!

NOW SHE UNDERSTANDS THE WHOLE ISSUE!

TRUDI'S WORK COMMENCED IN 2020 WHILST IN LOCKDOWN IN SPAIN BUT IT WAS HER RETURN TO JERSEY AND THE INSTIGATION OF WRITING AN 8-WEEK COURSE ON THE MENOPAUSE, THAT REALLY CEMENTED HER STEP INTO THE PERIMENOPAUSAL WORLD.

WWW.VITALITY40PLUS.COM
TRUDI@VITALITY40PLUS.COM

Chapter 23

SEX AND POO – BREAK THE TABOO!

By Trudi Roscouet

Ok, I bet you never thought this would be discussed in menopause. Well, that's what I do – break down those white walls – the barriers. Look, we could be affected by many symptoms, but having been an educator in menopause for the last couple of years, I wanted to share some of my secrets and insights on the things that no one wants to talk about!

So, who am I?

My name is Trudi from Jersey. I've worked in the corporate world for over 20 plus years. I'm a fully qualified adult teacher, A level 3 PT. I ran a gym where I specialised in women's and children's fitness and obesity. I took up boxing at the age of 45 years old. I've appeared in various TV programmes both Jersey, Spain and Gibraltar and been a guest of the Menopause Mandate in Parliament.

I'm now a fully-fledged menopause educator and wellbeing coach covering many of the offshore and crown dependencies.

My "interest" in menopause came from when I was about to leave Jersey for my new life in Spain in 2019.

I have an underactive thyroid, so I was about to set off on my journey when I discovered at the age of 51, I was in "the menopause".

Remembering the day vividly, I said to the female Doctor, "The WHAT?"

Roll on two years, Covid, Brexit, and whatever else could be thrown at me/us and we were locked down in Spain with no way to leave our apartment for over nine weeks. Hence, my own story into menopause research began. I knew the basics about weight loss – for god sake, I was a PT who specialised in women, so why was I struggling so very badly? That story will be for another day…

So here we are in 2023; I've been on HRT for 2.5 years and won't look back! But does that mean to say I am always swinging from a cloud – feeling as happy as larry (Who is larry, by the way!) and feeling fantastic? No, it does not! Anxiety is there creeping around, gnawing away at the pits of my stomach; my stomach can still bloat to look like I'm five months pregnant, and I suffer from extreme constipation! Yes, that's right, Like mega.

Not so much I don't go for days, but more my poo is very hard. I've always tended to be like this, even when I was younger.

Perhaps I should mention that I struggled with childhood anxiety due to parental divorce and breakup.

I was then diagnosed with Ulcerative Colitis and, later, IBS on top of the colitis. Colonoscopies and I were best friends (or not as the case may be) until I reached 40, when I was suddenly told I no longer had Ulcerative Colitis.

Fantastic, I thought – but then came the menopause. Oestrogen that once "assisted" the passing of poop down the track declines and, in my case, ceases. Therefore, the importance of increasing water supply is critical and I mean critical.

WARNING GRAPHIC ALERT, but when I don't drink sufficient water, it gets stuck and will tear the anal canal – commonly called fissures. Bleeding is likely. Hey, but no one warns you about constipation and solid stools!

So let's talk about SEX… or should I say vaginal dryness, soreness, itching, and add a touch of burning. Think of a nasty bout of thrush (those days when sex was fun!) and double it. Except it's not because you've just had a sex marathon but because declining oestrogen has dried up the tubes, and yet again, it starts with the vulva or what the doctors call vaginal atrophy where the skin becomes red and burning.

Working from home was a dream for many of us ladies. Skirts with no knickers and legs open to allow air to circulate – how Zoom could have made a fortune if full-length cameras had been invented.

But let's think of our front-line staff – nurses, teachers, childcare, paramedics etc. in uniforms. Not exactly the ideal scenario. Once the itching starts, it does not stop. You try to avoid it, but it takes control. Forget yoghurt; it's well past that! Then, the small tears begin to happen, and the pain increases. If left unattended, germs can seep up the tubes to cause Urinary Tract infections (UTIs). OK, I'll stop; there is no point in labouring at an already very tender point.

The good news is, ladies, there is something you can do about this straight away. Apart from female mutation, you can go immediately to a pharmacist, as from 2022, and ask for GINA – yup, that's right (VaGINA lol), and they will hand you pessaries. I made an urgent appointment with the Doctor, stating that this was a medical emergency, and he prescribed the cream Estradiol 1%. Pure bliss!

So, if this isn't enough for the final part of my chapter, it is the pure lack of sex drive.

I can hear the ladies sighing now, stating that with the above two things, why would you even consider wanting sex?

Of course, there should be a little thought to our beloved partners ?!?!? (or not??) How many ladies tell me, "Oh, the only symptom I have is losing my sex drive?"

This may not be critical to some couples, but I have seen and witnessed enough that men DO think this is an issue. We can tell by the divorce stats that there is a huge surge during 35-45 years (again, I am not putting this all down to the physical symptoms of menopause, you understand). Please, ladies, if this is an issue, do not ignore it. Once your oestrogen levels are under control, return to a doctor or specialist and talk Testosterone.

That's for another day.

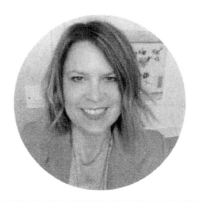

YVONNE DODD

YVONNE DODD HELPS WOMEN WHO ARE OVER 45 WITH LIMITING BELIEFS, TO LIVE THEIR UNIQUE LIVES BY DESIGN.

AFTER BECOMING FRUSTRATED AT TRYING TO FIT IN WITH SOMETIMES UNFAIR AND FRUSTRATING REGIMES AND FEELING LIKE THERE WERE CONSTRAINTS AROUND HER LIFE AND CHOICES,

YVONNE STARTED ON HER OWN SELF-DEVELOPMENT JOURNEY DELVING INTO NLP COACHING, HYPNOTHERAPY, MINDFULNESS TAPPING, AND SILENT COUNSELLING – ALL TRANSFORMATIVE MODALITIES THAT HEAL FROM THE CORE. YVONNE USED THESE TO TRANSFORM HER BELIEFS, AND NOW SHE HELPS OTHER WOMEN DO THE SAME.

YVONNEDODDCOACHING.CO.UK
YVONNEDODDCOACHING@GMAIL.COM

Chapter 24

HOW CAN YOU EMBRACE MENOPAUSE?

By Yvonne Dodd

Hi, my name is Yvonne, and at the time of writing this chapter, I'm 56 years old. Menopause has been relatively kind to me except for 'brain fog' and 'hot flushes', but I'm acutely aware of how debilitating it is for some women and the impact on their mental health and overall wellbeing.

I have been a Social Worker for 24 years and am a Mental Health Training Officer, and I have delivered training in my capacity as MHTO on menopause.

Around five years ago, I started a self-development journey, and during that time, I became a Neurolinguistic Programming Coach, Silent Counsellor, EFT and Mindfulness Practitioner and Hypnotherapist. I have been able to apply some of what I've learned to my personal experiences while working with women to help them achieve their goals.

Many women, but not all, are becoming empty nesters (I have mid-teens, started late at age 40) as their children are getting more independent and leaving home.

Or they are just saying, 'I've had enough of this,' and now it's time for me. For me, it combines spirituality, neuroscience, goal setting, energetics and health and wellbeing so that women have optimum informed choices about how to experience a better quality of life.

As menopause brings you to another metamorphic stage in your life, often women who have experienced trauma in their life, particularly during their teens, may experience debilitating symptoms when they start to go through menopause because this is the next big stage of the body making big changes in hormones and so it can evoke certain memories and emotions that have been buried within the subconscious mind. Often, this is due to the body holding on to a stagnant negative energy body that must be released and can impact your physical, mental and psychological wellbeing.

During menopause, there will be lots of ups and downs, so becoming more adaptable and resilient can make a difference in how you respond to obstacles that may come your way. How can you develop a growth mindset instead of a fixed mindset?

There is always a way to get out of your situation or how you feel.

If you haven't already thought about it, I'd like to introduce spirituality into your life to be more at peace and one with your body.

Don't forget your body has been there for you all your life, allowing you to breathe, have great life experiences, and possibly even give birth to another human.

Embrace the experiences and allow yourself to go through a journey of discovering the new you.

What can you do with your life now? There is a world of opportunities for you; you can sit and visualise the person you are about to become.

Your life does not need to end when you reach menopause, and starting something new like a new hobby, career, or business, go on a self-development and can open up a world of new opportunities for you.

If you allow yourself to do this; it can remove the focus from the symptoms that may not feel good for you.

Ask yourself how to break free from limiting beliefs and think of it as an opportunity to shed old skin and rejuvenate with a new you, purpose, clarity and perspective. Embrace your knowledge, skills and experience and believe in your capacity to do whatever you want. Only you can change what is for you and how you feel inside. Think of menopause as a time of self-reflection and listening to your body more.

When I work with women, I use muscle testing because the body has all the answers; it knows everything, and we should listen to it more. It also possesses the power to intuitively know when something is right or wrong because everything is made of energy.

If you want to increase your energy, feel more fulfilled and have more fun in life, think about what lights you up so you can become more energetically aligned with the future. Can you do more of that? How often can you implement practices into your life? Can you put it into your diary to ensure you look after yourself more often? As women, we generally take on caring roles and responsibilities and feel guilty when doing something for ourselves. It's time to change that because self-care isn't selfish; it's about ensuring you look after your wellbeing so your health doesn't decline.

Our brains are made of neuroplasticity, so at any time, we can change the neurons in our brain to rewire by practising many different techniques and strategies and changing our daily habits, leading to a new, improved identity.

What new opportunities can you look out for? How can you improve your life by owning your mental, physical and spiritual health?

Start meditation by allowing your thoughts to come and go; it takes a lot of practice and the realisation that thoughts will always be there, but observe them like you are a third party with no judgement. You can also practice box breathing, allowing the central nervous to calm down when overthinking or anxiety occurs. Breathe deeply for 5, hold for five and breathe out for 5. This allows your mind to rest because when you focus on breathing, your mind cannot wander.

Embrace yourself and who you are; you are unique and have many qualities and life experiences. You can take your power back and control how your mind and body work instead of it controlling you.

Epilogue

We hope you've enjoyed reading this book and have taken a lot from it in order to help you navigate your way through your own menopause journey.

If you're not there yet, let this book be a guide on what you can do to prepare yourself to make your path easier in the years to come.

It's never too late to start exercising, eating right or meditating, so if you've read this and thought, I'm nearly at the end or I'm over it now, you can always improve your lifestyle at any age.

Menopause symptoms can last for many years after your last period and so it's important to be aware or the strategies you can put in place before, during and after. This book will help you do that.

If you'd like to be involved in sharing your own menopause journey or any strategies you may have to help others, please do get in touch with The Book Chief at thebookchief.com

References

Chapter 20

Dimitrov, S., Hulteng, E., & Hong, S. (2017). Inflammation and exercise: Inhibition of monocytic intracellular TNF production by acute exercise via β2-adrenergic activation. Brain, Behavior, and Immunity, 61, 60-68. Retrieved from https://doi.org/10.1016/j.bbi.2016.12.017.

Woods, J.A., Wilund, K.R., Martin, S.A., & Kistler, B.M. (2012). Exercise, inflammation and ageing. Aging & Disease, 3(1), 130-140. Retrieved from https://www.ncbi.nlm.nih.gov/pmc/articles/PMC3320801/

Chapter 21

Bonanno, G.A., Romero, S.A., & Klein, S.I. (2015). The Temporal Elements of Psychological Resilience: An Integrative Framework for the Study of Individuals, Families, and Communities. Psychological Inquiry, 26(2), 139–169. https://doi.org/10.1080/1047840X.2015.992677.

Süss, H., Willi, J., Grub, J., & Ehlert, U. (2020). Psychosocial factors promoting resilience during the menopausal transition. Archives of Women's Mental Health, 24(2), 231–241. https://doi.org/10.1007/s00737-020-01055-7.

Thomas, A.J., Mitchell, E.S., & Woods, N.F. (2018). The challenges of midlife women: themes from the Seattle midlife Women's health study. Women's Midlife Health, 4(1). https://doi.org/10.1186/s40695-018-0039-9.

About the Creator of this book

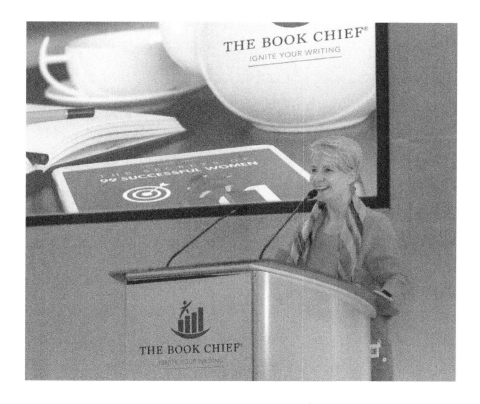

SHARON BROWN moved to the West Midlands in 2003 from Glasgow in Scotland. After a wide-ranging career in Event Management, Marketing, Project Management and board level support in various industries, Sharon started an Events Agency in 2015 which has grown into the Award-winning Lydian Group Ltd.

After realising that business was heading more towards the online digital space, Sharon launched four online platforms, the first being a Women in Business platform in 2018 with a mission of creating 'Collaboration over Competition'.

Two further projects were launched during lockdown with the aim of helping small business owners build their brands through speaking, writing, publishing, and collaborative working. MO2VATE Magazine was born in 6 weeks from concept to implementation and received a fantastic following through its subscribers and supporters. It's now seeing a complete facelift this year ready for its relaunch as MO2VATE Media, seeing it evolve as a membership driven business and information hub.

The Speakers Index was the third platform to be launched as Sharon saw a gap in the market around Speaking Agencies and the lack of promotion towards their speakers. The Speakers Index is an online directory which also houses a quality Speakers Magazine highlighting the speakers' talents. Members are encouraged to create a full profile giving all the information needed by an Organiser who can then contact them directly through their contact details on the website or in the magazine.

The Book Chief is Sharon's Award-winning publishing house, launched in 2021, already with an impressive resume of clients and Authors.

Sharon's vision was to provide an all-in-one affordable publishing service turning small business owners into credible authors through a robust and structured process and collaborative partners. The Book Chief portfolio has exponentially grown during the past two years and continues to build huge momentum both in the UK and with overseas clients.

Services

The Book Chief Publishing House

The Book Chief Publishing House was born during the latter end of the pandemic with a mission to support business owners on their path to becoming credible Authors.

The Book Chief publishes every genre, type and size of book and advises on every step of producing your book from book covers, titles, book descriptions, your best chance to become a best-selling Author and much more.

The Book Chief has a great track record in customer service and of producing great results for your book both in layout, editing, design and marketing.

As a one-stop shop for all your Publishing needs, and payment plans to spread the cost, it should be the first stop for those looking to publish and spread the word about their book!

Thebookchief.com

sharon@thebookchief.com

MO2VATE Media

MO2VATE is a global digital business hub covering topics across business industries, health, inspiration, lifestyle, politics, opinion / research-based information, entrepreneur insights and many other topics, founded by Sharon Brown.

Formerly known as MO2VATE Magazine, this new platform launches in November 2022 with a completely new concept to share important information globally.

All articles are written by business owners and the project is managed by independent entrepreneurs. The online hub runs yearly International Awards and produces various books written by the Contributors who are part of the MO2VATE community.

Mo2vatemedia.com

editor@mo2vatemagazine.com

The Speakers Index

The Speakers Index is an online directory for speakers and event organisers designed to improve their chances of being seen by the right people.

We produce a quarterly magazine where each speaker features on a double page spread. The magazine is sent out through social media and to our email list on each publication.

Working similar to an agency but without any additional fees or commission, The Speakers Index also creates events to allow speakers to participate and be seen.

Thespeakersindex.com

sharon@thespeakersindex.com